Losing It—
NATURALLY

Also by Loretta Washburn

Book

*Mind Travelers:
Portraits of Famous Psychics
and Healers of Today*

Audiocassette

*The Practical Art of Magick:
Creating Your Own Path*

LORETTA WASHBURN

Losing It— NATURALLY

A Complete Holistic Weight Loss Program

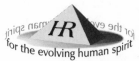

HAMPTON ROADS
PUBLISHING COMPANY, INC.

Copyright © 1999
by Loretta Washburn

All rights reserved, including the right to reproduce this
work in any form whatsoever, without permission
in writing from the publisher, except for brief passages
in connection with a review.

Cover design by Marjoram Productions
Cover photography by
Jacque Denzer Parker, Indexstock Photography
Peter Johansky, Indexstock Photography
Ewing Galloway, Indexstock Photography
Dave Bartruff, Indexstock Photography
Tom Ross, Indexstock Photography
Fred Slavin, Indexstock Photography
Interior art by David Brown

For information write:

Hampton Roads Publishing Company, Inc.
134 Burgess Lane
Charlottesville, VA 22902

Or call: 804-296-2772
FAX: 804-296-5096
e-mail: hrpc@hrpub.com
Web site: http://www.hrpub.com

If you are unable to order this book from your local
bookseller, you may order directly from the publisher.
Quantity discounts for organizations are available.
Call 1-800-766-8009, toll-free.

Library of Congress Catalog Card Number: 98-73917

ISBN 1-57174-122-4

10 9 8 7 6 5 4 3 2 1

Printed on acid-free recycled paper in Canada

Dedication

This book is dedicated to all of you who want to live a life that is never stuck or static or stale, who want every moment to be new and fresh. For those who choose to take the power of their own mind and create their own circumstances.

Disclaimer

Table of Contents

acknowledgements

I want to offer my heartfelt thanks to Bob Friedman, publisher of Hampton Roads Publishing Company, Inc. for asking me to write this book. Thank you for believing in me and for your patience, as I did not always meet deadlines. I also want to thank everyone on your staff that helped pull this book together. I want to thank Hampton Roads Publishing Company, Inc., editorial staff for their hard work, especially Rebecca Williamson for applying those invaluable final touches to this manuscript to help make it the book I had hoped it would be. You did it under a very tight deadline and did it with an enthusiastic spirit. I thank Marjoram Productions, Jonathan and Matthew Friedman, for giving me a beautiful book cover; you gave me exactly what I asked for. Jane Hagaman, the art director, did a great job with handling the interior art and keeping me updated with the completion of the book.

I want to offer a very special thanks to William Crook, M.D., of Jackson, Tennessee, author of *The Yeast Connection Handbook—1999*, for allowing me the use of the *Candida albicans* questionnaire in my book. I would also like to thank you for all of the information that you provided for me to help make this a great book. You have educated and helped thousands of people with their yeast-related problems. I honor you.

Robert Crayhon, nutritionist and author of *The Carnitine Miracle*, requires a very special thank you, as you gave me all of the help that I needed in reference to carnitine and kept me supplied with carnitine to help me stay mentally alert and give me energy, which made the writing of this book much easier.

I would like to thank David Christopher, president of Christopher Publications, for allowing me to use excerpts from his father's book, *Dr. Christopher's 3 Day Cleansing Program, Mucusless Diet and Herbal Combination*.

I gratefully thank Dr. Donald Papon, author of *Homeopathy Made Simple*, for your dedication to teach us to heal the planet. You are awesome. Thank you for your friendship and for keeping me healthy!

I would also like to thank all of my family and friends who understood the privacy and support that I needed while writing this book. A very special thank you to my very cool and fabulous daughters Shelly Peabody, Heidi Fruchtenicht, and Gerda Gartner. Thank you to my grandson, Mark Gartner. You are the greatest! You are just a little boy and you understood that you could not spend as much time with me while I wrote this book. It's great being your Honey.

Thank you to sweet Bob Nielsen. You gave me so much of your valuable time and help. You encouraged me when I was feeling low; you brought me up, you were there for everything that I needed. Without you I could not have completed the book as smoothly as I did and I thank you for being in my life.

I also thank my brother Louis Schlosser. Though growing up in a very dysfunctional family, you always made sure that I knew that I was loved. I would also like to thank my mother, Lois Schlosser, who taught me to finish what I start.

introduction

How many of you have dieted unsuccessfully? Maybe you've dieted not once, not twice, but maybe for a lifetime, starving yourself or drinking some awful shake, to find it worked only temporarily. You lose ten pounds, taking three to four weeks to accomplish this, and in one short weekend, you've gained it all back.

I think that we have all been there, done that. Dieting simply does not work.

I'm going to teach you the things that do work. You're going to find out why you have gained weight, or have always been packing around that extra poundage. (Most people try to lose weight without trying to figure out why they are carrying around the extra weight.)

Excessive weight signals that your body is lacking something, or something within is simply out of balance. Or, your thought patterns may need an adjustment—you are and will be whatever it is that you believe you are. So, if you think you're fat, you will be exactly that. I believe it was Albert Einstein who said that imagination was more important than knowledge.

We look at someone who is overweight and assume that person spends all of his or her time eating, when in fact this person may not eat any more than a thin person. We'll find out why one overeats and we'll teach you and give you wonderful tips on how to curb your appetite. Through different types of self-testing, you will figure it out.

It's my intention to help you to slim down and be healthier as gently and easily as I can. I want you to live longer, be happier, love yourself, and live every day with great passion. I want you to be healthy and feel young, look young, and have the energy that you should have.

I'm going to make it as easy on you as I can. Depending on your problem, it may take a lot of work and some time, but the results will indeed be worth it. I want to promote natural weight loss, to promote energy. I include exercise to help you build muscle and tone your body. Exercise will also stimulate and promote weight loss quicker and more efficiently. The exercises that you will be doing are gentle on your body, and I'm not expecting you to do anything that I wouldn't do. I certainly do not like spending a great deal of time exercising. If things are too much, I tend to lose motivation.

You also need to keep in mind that before you make any big changes involving your health, always check with your physician and let him or her know what it is that you are wanting to do. If you have any serious health problems, your doctor needs to okay any changes that you are making. This is very important!

You have the right to choose alternative methods of being healthier over modern medicine, or combine methods. It's time for you to make a choice. Vitamins are immeasurably safer than drugs; you decide—you are paying the bill. Keep in mind that no one cares as much about you as you, and you owe it to yourself to know as much about your health as you possibly can.

chapter 1

my story

Growing up, I was always a little bit round. I guess saying round sounds a whole lot better than saying fat. Of
course it was my brothers and sisters who called me fat,
not to mention ugly, stupid, and whatever else they could
think of. Children are so cruel. Then there was my dad,
who always told me that I wasn't fat, that I was prettier
than the bee's knees. Parents always think their little girls
are beautiful.

My body simply did what all children's bodies do. Before you go through a growing spurt, it seems like you
kind of plump up a bit, then stretch up in height as you
grow. At age ten I was close to the height I am now, and
suddenly as skinny as a rail. This was a benefit to me, as I
had the opportunity at age fifteen to do a little modeling. I
could eat and eat and never gain any weight. I remember
my mother telling me to slow down with my eating because
it would catch up with me someday. I would come home
from school and eat as many as five peanut butter and jelly
sandwiches. It didn't catch up with me. I stayed skinny,

13

not to mention depressed, and exhibited many other symptoms of problems, but I didn't know any better because I had never felt any other way. It was simply a part of me.

Much later, I started getting symptoms of other problems. I had a degenerative disease in my spine, bursitis in my hips; the eating had finally caught up with me and I was overweight, and felt like an old woman. I was old before my time. There were chiropractors and physical therapists I was seeing on a regular basis. I was in pain every breathing moment.

Then things began to change. I approached Hampton Roads Publishing with my first book, *Mind Travelers: Portraits of Famous Psychics and Healers of Today*. They wanted the book. Writing that book was one of the most important things that I had ever done for myself. If you can, imagine thirty very gifted people healing you in one form or another. Thirty people in a two-year period—that's a lot of hands-on healing.

I had gone to New York City to photograph and interview Robert Zoller, a very well-known astrologer, who asked me if I also wanted to have Dr. R. Donald Papon, who is a doctor of homeopathic medicine, in my book. I was thrilled to think of including the man who is considered the dean of astrology. I had bought my first book of his in 1976. It was his dream book, which I have used so much that I have a rubber band around it to keep it together. Dr. Papon agreed to participate in my book and I drove up to Princeton from Virginia Beach to meet with him.

After returning home from meeting with him, I sent him a thank-you note for being a part of my book and being so kind to me. His return letter came with a package filled with homeopathic remedies. He had analyzed my health and concluded that I was a mess. I weighed 162 pounds. I might add that I was very uncomfortable in my skin.

The remedies were for many things. My thyroid wasn't working; there was a remedy for that. I had *Candida*; there was another remedy. There was also a remedy for parasites he found in my system, which were partly responsible for my bloated belly. My blood sugar was also down.

I had remedies in that package for everything. Those remedies, little white pills that are placed under the tongue to dissolve, would cure these ailments. I must admit, I had very little faith in this. However, I followed the doctor's advice to the T—I figured I wouldn't know if all this would work unless I gave it my best shot.

I had to go on a very strict diet to get rid of the *Candida*, which is yeast. So, any food or drink that feeds yeast, I had to eliminate from my diet. Now this wasn't a diet to lose weight; it was a diet to kill off the yeast in my system. This meant no sugar, no processed foods, yeast, vinegar, mushrooms, wine, or caffeine. I thought this diet would be impossible for me, but my desire to be healthy and to lose weight outweighed the desire to have some sugar. When you tell yourself that you can't have something *right now*, it's very easy for your mind to let go of wanting it. It wasn't bad at all. Three months later I had melted down to one hundred twelve pounds. I started out at one sixty-two. I had been wearing a junior size fifteen, which was too small for me; I managed to pour myself into those jeans. Most people had no idea that I weighed that much because I wore baggy tops.

After the diet, I had gone down to a size five. My skin felt so good. I felt as though I had let go of another person, that there had been someone else in that skin with me.

I had been depressed for years, only I didn't even know it until I was no longer in that state. I couldn't make decisions easily; I would get confused easily, not being able to focus my mind on one thing for very long. My nails would crack and tear very easily and my hair was dry. My skin itched many times, as though something were crawling beneath it. My relationships were never very secure feeling; when things got bad, I would bail out. Well, I needed to bail, because I would make bad choices. I also had times of suicidal tendencies.

And there were the cravings for sugar, especially chocolate. Did I love chocolate—yet the state I'm in today, I couldn't care less about the stuff. With the *Candida*, sugars feed it, so you crave what it is that your body wants. Not that my body itself wanted the chocolate; the yeast in my system wanted it.

You will also crave what you are allergic to, and eating what you are allergic to will make you gain weight.

There is so much about our health, about our diets, that we are never taught. I am hoping that through this book you will learn about your body and how to take care of it. Your body is a temple; honor it. People take better care of their automobiles than they do their own instrument, themselves.

All the symptoms I was referring to earlier are symptoms of hypothyroidism, *Candida albicans,* parasites, allergies, and hypoglycemia, which is low blood sugar. Maybe you have no energy, you tire easily, you are hungry all the time, and you cannot lose weight. You could starve yourself and the weight would still be there, hanging on for dear life, or so it seems.

You may have some of these symptoms, more than likely you have one or two, maybe more of these conditions that I am speaking about. We are going to get you straight and keep you there. This book isn't just about losing weight; it's about being healthy and taking great care of yourself.

I had gone through the homeopathic remedies, as I said, and lost fifty pounds in just a few short months. It was absolutely the best. It was as if I had found myself, as if I had myself back. Not only did I look terrific, I was no longer depressed or confused; I could make decisions without getting upset.

The weight stayed off me for four years, and it was easy. Killing off the yeast was tough because of the diet that I had to stick to in a very strict manner, but it was well worth it.

Last year was a bit tough. I had become very ill; the doctors said that I had bronchitis. After three months of this illness, with a serious cough and only getting worse, I finally consulted my homeopath, Dr. Papon. I felt as though I were dying, and I had plumped up and couldn't lose the weight.

According to Dr. Papon, I had mercury poisoning. I'm also a photographer, and got the poisoning from the chemicals that I was using. The mercury poisoning had thrown my system off and again I had *Candida*. Dr. Papon sent some remedies off to me, giving me gold as an antidote and, of course, something for the yeast.

Within a week, I was feeling good again. The weight melted off easily and stayed off until I took a trip to Europe. The food there was out of this world and I ate and ate. I gained weight, but it wasn't because I was eating too much; I had picked up a parasite.

I was in Europe for two months, a long time, going from country to country. I tried to be very careful, but I couldn't stay away from the water, or I may have picked up the parasites from the food. When I got home, I knew that I had picked up these little pests; my belly was bloated and I simply had all the symptoms.

This time I decided to take care of this on my own. I started eating garlic, and as a backup, I took some black walnut extract. An entire clove of garlic—pure, straight, chunka-chunka garlic—became a part of my daily routine. I peeled it off, cut the ends off, peeled it down, and popped it into my mouth with a glass of water at hand to wash it down. Not a pleasant taste, but I know that it is incredibly good for me for many things and will kill the critters that I do not want to carry around with me. The garlic I simply take every day and will continue to take for a great long time.

And, do I smell like garlic? No! I never do. So often when someone eats garlic, it seems to exude from his or her pores. It does not happen to me; I don't want to smell like garlic, so—it is my intention to not have that smell about me.

One of the things that I teach is to create your own reality; the power of the mind is fascinating. I tell the universe what it is that I am choosing and the universe provides. We are all incredible manifesters, and I practice what I preach. You can learn all about creating your own reality through my tapes, *The Practical Art of Magick*.

Stress is another factor in gaining weight. Through eating in a more healthy way, getting all the nutrients that we need and a good exercise program, we can stay healthy, stress-free, and even young for a very long time. It is my intention to stay young. And what that means to me is feeling youthful, being able to do all the physical things that I want and need to do. I want to move without pain; as a little vanity steps in, I want to keep the figure that I have for a very long time. I enjoy the fact that people often think that I'm about fifteen years younger than I really am. Not that I give them that impression by lying about my age. I'm quite proud that I'm forty-seven, and don't look old enough to be a grandmother (although my grandson refers to me as "Honey" rather than "Grandma"). He came up with the name on his own with no coaxing. There I go being a typical grandmother, talking about my grandson, as if he has something to do with weight loss. However, chasing him around doesn't hurt.

Besides the garlic that I eat, which I believe is much more potent that garlic pills, there are many other things that I do to stay in shape, which I'm not going to go into right now. You'll learn about these things as we go further into the book.

There is one other thing that I do want to discuss with you here. I do drink a great deal of water. I drink bottled spring water. I go through about a gallon every two days. I drink it with lemon; we need a great deal of citrus in our system. Most people don't get near enough citrus in their diets. I also drink seltzer water with lemon wedges.

Water is good for you for many reasons, one of my favorite reasons is what water has done for me, in the visual sense. I started getting wrinkles at a very young age and my hands have never been pretty. My hands, in the past, have looked like an old woman's hands. That was always disturbing to me. I would straighten my hand out, stretch my fingers out and the skin on the top of my hands would wrinkle up, scrunch up, and look like crinkly paper. Ugly! A female friend of mine, Kathy Oddenino, who is in my book *Mind Travelers*, writes beautiful books on healing yourself through proper nutrition. One of the things that she taught me was to drink lots of water, and it would aid in my wrinkles, and my crinkly-skinned hands. Well, it worked and is still working, because I will continue to drink as much water as I can. Even the texture of my skin has improved, and is much softer than it has ever been.

The way our skin looks is a big factor in showing our age. I realize that this book is about ridding yourself of unwanted pounds; however, I also want to teach you how to be healthier and feel good. If you look good, you are probably going to also be feeling pretty good. It all works together.

I haven't told you that this is necessarily going to be all that easy. For some of you, it might; some of you may have to work a little bit harder. I'm assuming that you bought this book because you want to do something about your weight and your health; you know the two go hand in hand. Along with getting yourself where it is that you want to be, we also need to work on your body; get your body into motion. Get up and move! You can speed up the weight loss up by getting physical. This doesn't mean that you have to go and join a gym. You can be gentle on your body, and yet very effective. Often it is hard to exercise alone; maybe you need support to keep you motivated.

A few years ago I decided that I would get out and walk every morning or evening; I would do it for a while then stop. I wanted it to be a natural thing and I wanted to incorporate this into my life where it would be a habit; I would have no resistance to it. Well, I would walk and then I wouldn't walk. Keep in mind that going out and taking a stroll is not going to do you much good. You want to walk with passion, walk fast, no—speed it up, walk even faster. What I decided to do was to get one of my daughters to go out and do this with me. Sometimes I would get lucky and I would have the company of two of my daughters going with me. They could never keep up with me; I meant business; I wanted to walk and get my blood flowing, moving, work up a good healthy sweat. I only walk for twenty minutes. That's not very long, but it works.

I failed to mention how I walk, or rather where. I found that if I were to plan to get up and just head out the door to walk, I was less apt to do it. So, I began to get up early in the morning, get ready, and drive down to the beach, park my car, and walk on the boardwalk. It was only fifteen minutes from my house and a beautiful place to be. That's something that you may want to consider trying if there is a park near where you are living, or a walking trail, or maybe you, too, live near the beach or someplace equally as beautiful. Don't forget to do some stretching before you go out there and start pounding your hoofies on the ground.

I talk about this in the past tense because I have recently moved to downtown Norfolk. Before, I was in Virginia Beach, which made it much easier to get down to the boardwalk. I'm not that much farther away, but it's not something I really want to be doing. I have found something even better that works for me. I have recently adopted a beautiful Rottweiler. He used to belong to my daughter. Zeus was living in a very small apartment with not a great deal of attention; not that my daughter was a bad dog owner; she just spends a lot of time with her work.

Well, I was thrilled to take him, and he is now my walking partner. We get up early in the morning and go for our walk. It took a while to get him used to this whole speed-walking thing. At first he would wrap around my legs, stop and sniff the grass where all the other dogs had stopped to do whatever, and take off in other directions. I hung in there with him and he now gets the picture. He loves it and we both get our exercise. The walk has changed; we now go out every morning and every evening to walk. I'm not saying that you have to do this twice a day, but if you can take twenty minutes to go out and walk, and walk as quickly as you can, the benefits will be astounding. This will be a wonderful addition to the other things you are doing to lose weight.

I'm by all means not an exercise freak; I am a "let's be healthy" freak. I want to be trim, but I don't necessarily want to be hurting; I think that exercise should be gentle. I don't want to be muscle bound; I kind of like my round curves and degree of softness. I also believe that men prefer a woman with curves. What's most important is that I like myself the way I am.

I do other exercises besides walking. What I am most concerned with, as most women are, is my butt and my thighs. I can get down on the floor and do all kinds of exercises, and every once in a while I do. I don't go to a gym; I don't have time for it. However, gyms are great and if you find them also to be a great place to meet health-minded people, make new friends or whatever, do whatever makes you happy. I simply prefer to keep my exercising private.

Now I'm going to tell you what it is that I do—don't laugh! Every evening when I'm winding down, I open my closet and pull out two little tools. Oh yes, with these tools, you'll never have to back out of a room naked again. Some of you are wondering, what? Why would someone have to back out of a room? Then there are those of you who know exactly what I'm talking about. Have you ever been naked with your partner and you had to leave the room, to go to the bathroom, the kitchen, or wherever? Maybe you were getting creative and just made love on the dining room table, in the pantry, or on top of the washing machine!

You find yourself walking backward, saying, "Baby, please don't look at my butt." As crazy as that may sound or seem, I have done that more times than I would like to admit. I've been naked and walked out of the bedroom, backward with my hand out, looking like The Supremes singing "Stop! In the Name of Love." Got the picture? Then there's the walk slowly deal so that the butt doesn't move too much.

I have gotten away from that, thanks to Suzanne Somers. Yes, I'm talking about the Masters—the Butt Master and the Thigh Master. Are you laughing? You shouldn't! Let me tell you, a week after using the Butt Master, my heinie lifted and became much firmer. There was a time when I never worried too much about it, figuring that it was behind me and what I couldn't see, couldn't hurt. Wrong!

I actually bought the Thigh Master first. It was great and smoothed out my thighs, very quickly too, I might add. I wasn't really all that big, just not firm. Then when the Butt Master came out, I thought maybe this tool, or piece of equipment, would be just as good as its sister piece of equipment. Maybe I could stop walking backward out of a room.

I pull the Masters out every night and use them for firming up. You can also use the Thigh Master for your arms. I have found that my stomach is also in better shape from using these tools. I started off with squeezing twenty times and worked my way up to one hundred. I highly recommend it. It's easy, it's gentle, and it works.

You should also make it fun. Life in general should be fun. When I'm doing my exercises, I chant, I sing, I make up songs, and just make it enjoyable. I sing things like, of course there has to be a rhythm to it, okay, here we go,

"My butt, my butt, I feel it getting smaller, it's tight, it's tight, I feel it getting tighter—oh yes, oh yes, it burns a little, but it's going to look better!" Just go on and on, as silly as it sounds. It makes it fun and I'm also making positive statements about how I'm looking.

I'm sure that my butt wasn't as bad as I believed it was. When you grow up with comments from your brother, those things stick in your mind. Of course he made his comments as I was walking out of a room. He would say things like, "Stop for a minute. It's amazing how when you stop, your butt is still moving." My brother was just teasing me, but it took years to let go of those thought patterns. By the way, we will also be working on the way you think and feel about yourself.

Thought is energy and energy creates energy. The spoken word is the same. It is energy and we are whatever it is we believe we are. If you say things such as, "I'm fat and I will always be fat," or anything similar, you are what you believe you are, and you become what you believe you are. Start changing your thought patterns; choose the words that you use more carefully. Look in the mirror and make statements that you can become in harmony with. Say things like "I'm beautiful, I like the way I am looking. I am getting thinner. It is easy for me to lose the weight that I want to lose." Positive reinforcement is very powerful and a very wise thing to do. We'll get into that more along the way.

chapter 2

laura

I want to share with you my experience with meeting and spending time with a beautiful lady, Laura. I went to Sedona, Arizona, a year ago to do some research for another book that I am writing. Laura invited me to stay with her for the four days that I would be there. Her house was right on one of the earth vortexes. I knew that I would have some wonderful experiences sitting in the energy of Cathedral Rock.

Needless to say, I did very little work on my book. I was too busy doing research on this lady. I watched her, studied her, and picked her brain. I'm telling you about her because she was such an inspiration to me. She is in her mid-seventies, married to a gorgeous man in his thirties. Did I mention that she, too, is gorgeous? This is a woman with the body of a woman in her twenties. In fact, she puts most women in their twenties to shame. She had *no* wrinkles, *no* cellulite, *no* stretch marks, and the list goes on and on. I had to find out what this woman does to keep young.

25

I found that her intention is to stay young and beautiful and to live until forever. It sounded good to me, and I'm always looking for a new way to be healthier and defy aging. Not that aging is a bad thing; I'm simply in no big hurry to move along in that direction.

The first night there was kind of rough on me. I had just driven from Virginia to California to do some seminars at a whole life expo. From there, I drove back down to Arizona, all in the company of my two-year-old grandson. This made for an intense trip. My first night there, I didn't really spend any time with Laura. I just wanted to sleep.

The following day I went out exploring and tried my darnedest to do my research, but all I could think about was this woman and how she looked. That night, I told her I wanted her to share it all with me. Why didn't she have any wrinkles and why was she in such great shape? I wanted to know everything about her so I could do whatever it was that she was doing. I would like to stay young looking without going under the knife. If it can be done naturally, I want to know all about it. We stayed up until three o'clock in the morning for the next three nights and she spent every breathing moment teaching me all of her secrets. I feel that it is very important for me to share all the information with you. I know you, too, will want to know all about this woman.

First, I asked her about her hands and face. Her hands were like that of a young girl, and there were no lines on her face.

She took a good look at my hand. I was a bit embarrassed; this woman was about thirty years older than me and her hands looked better than mine. She talked about the dryness of my skin and how thirsty it must be. If I took better care of it, it would change, she said. Her advice was lotion—she told me to feed my skin. I think common sense tells you that if you moisturize your skin, of course it will be in better shape, but it's very easy to neglect the little things, like putting lotion on your skin. She had me lotioning my entire body, for more reasons than just feeding my crocodile skin. The rubbing and massaging get the circulation going and are also great for breaking up cellulite.

I asked her about the crinkly skin on the top of my hands. She told me to start pinching the skin—not real hard, but pinch and pinch and pinch some more. This would get the circulation going and the skin would become more taut. It sounded crazy to me, but I also knew that this was indeed a wise woman and I would indeed follow her directions.

You don't know if something is actually going to work unless you try it. I'm open to new ideas. So, I pinched and pinched some more. I pinched the top of my hands and around my eyes, wherever I had lines on my face. Remember, you do this in a very gentle manner. I don't want you to be bruising yourself or damaging your skin in any way. The amazing thing was that it worked. I moisturized my face and the tops of my hands, and began my gentle pinching; in just a couple of short weeks, there truly was a difference.

Like me, Laura approaches her health in a holistic way. We need to find natural ways of healing ourselves. Illness and disease are caused from the lack of proper nutrition, and I believe you can heal every illness, whether it is an emotional or a physical illness, through proper nutrition. I also believe that to be healthy we need to be in balance in body, mind, and spirit.

Okay, I had the wrinkle thing covered, now—what about this woman's body, the shape that she was in? One of the things that she does every night, which I think is very important, is give herself a foot and hand massage. She does reflexology on her hands and feet. I also do this—it will keep your body in fine tune.

On the palms of your hands and the bottoms of your feet, there are pressure points that control all of your organs. You can fix all your aches and pains and balance your body, from getting rid of headaches to taking care of constipation.

When you are just sitting and watching television, or just being still, start feeling the palms of your hands. Take your thumb and rub and press your opposite hand. Push your thumb on every area of the palm of your hand and down your fingers, covering the entire inside part of your hand and fingers. When you press, and there is a sore spot, continue pressing and releasing over and over until it no longer hurts. By pressing, you are releasing the block of that particular part of your body that is being controlled.

Go down to your feet and do the same thing. When you find a sore spot, work on it until it releases and is no longer sore. This can be very uncomfortable; at the same time, you will be helping to balance your body. You may find that you will stop having headaches, sinus infections, or other health problems.

Laura does this every night. When she finds a sore spot, she eliminates it immediately, and it seems to keep her very agile. One night, she was lying on the floor of her living room, reached down, wrapped her hand around her ankle, and lifted her leg up along the side of her head. She doesn't go out and work out, she simply lies on her living room floor every night and does a few exercises, mostly just stretches.

She says that people get old because they stop moving their bodies. She does some toe touches and lies on the floor to do some leg lifts from the side and the back, some sit-ups, and she is done.

She also believes that she's young and healthy. You know, we are what we believe we are. I've watched her movements, her actions, as she hops in and out of her Jeep. She hasn't an ache or pain in her body, and everything she does, she does with passion. I believe that life should be filled with passion. You should feel passion in loving, passion for your work. In everything you do, do it with great passion. If you don't feel passion in your life, start making yourself happy. When you follow your bliss, the passion will follow. I hope that my story about Laura may have inspired you; she most definitely made a huge impact on my life. I hope that when I'm in my seventies, my body is as fluid as hers. Oh, to capture longevity!

chapter 3

homeopathy and weight loss

I shared with you earlier my introduction to homeopathy through Dr. Donald Papon. While I recommend it, I don't feel that you should try to do the homeopathy on your own. If this is the avenue you choose to lose your weight, find a good homeopathic physician and let him or her take care of you.

I think one of the most important things that needs to be addressed is the psychological aspect. Often we gain weight when we have emotional stuff going on. This is where the "Each" remedies can help very much. Each remedies are another system of healing, a system of herbal remedies. These are usually dispensed in tincture or liquid form, according to the dominant mental state or states of the patient. These floral remedies alter disharmonies in the emotional states and personality that, if left untreated, eventually cause physical illness.

Dr. Papon also works with the Each remedies along with his homeopathic work. He says that an example of an Each remedy is crabapple, which helps with self-worth. When we gain weight, our self-worth goes down. When we want to lose weight, we have to look at the needs of the total person.

People often say that they can't change things that are going on in their lives. You can change anything; start with the things that you feel that you can change. Gaining weight is the body saying to you, "Pay attention to me." One of the problems is that people simply give up. The answer is not to give up, but to get up. Get up and do something about your life; make some changes; make yourself number one; love yourself. I don't mean this in an arrogant way, but start putting yourself in the number one place.

Dr. Papon feels that it isn't just so much what you are eating, but how much you are eating; it's a number game. He feels that there is a connection between what you are eating and when you are eating it. For example, your main meal maybe should be at lunch time and then you can have something light for dinner, such as a salad. Everyone's body is different; you want to experiment with your meals to find out what works best for you.

We are also becoming more sedentary. Our children are coming home from school and planting themselves in front of the television or are becoming glued to the computer. We are teaching our children to sit; we have to get them up and moving around. Children are becoming less and less involved in outdoor sports, or even just going outside and playing. They want to be in front of the computer to play games.

I think in general this problem affects everyone, not just the children. When I was young, I was forced to go outside and get fresh air. (Maybe not so forced, I wanted to be outdoors.) Maybe my mother just wanted me out of her hair, and again maybe she felt that I needed to be outdoors, running and playing, breathing in the fresh air. We have to get our children and ourselves up and moving around.

WHAT IS HOMEOPATHY?

Homeopathy is a system of energy healing using minute amounts of safe, nontoxic, natural substances derived from the vegetable, animal, and mineral kingdoms, dispensed from the "Law of Similars"—an age-old principle that recognizes the body's ability to heal itself.

The word "homeopathy" is derived from the Greek, and means "like suffering." So, a homeopath treats like with like, similar to a vaccine.

Homeopathy goes way back, has been expounded by Hindu medical manuscripts, recognized by Aristotle, applied by Hippocrates, and further endorsed by other famous medieval physicians.

Christian Samuel Hahnemann rediscovered homeopathy a couple hundred years ago. Hahnemann found 99 remedies; today there is a list of over 2000 different remedies. I have heard many times that you cannot take more than one remedy at a time because they will counteract one another, and many practitioners agree with this. However, Dr. Papon believes that this is not true. He says that you can take more than one if you just do not mix them in your mouth at one time. The little pills are put under your tongue and held there until they dissolve, which happens immediately. Following one, you can then take another, and another. It is also said that you cannot touch these pills with your fingers, which also is not true. It is also often said that you cannot take allopathic drugs (drugs from a regular physician) while taking homeopathic remedies. This is also not true. You simply take any kind of medication that you may need at a different time of the day from when you take your remedies so that you are not taking them together.

Homeopathy is practiced all over the world. In France, according to Dr. Papon, there are five homeopathic physicians to each allopathic physician. There, as you can see, the preferred choice of health care is the natural way.

Homeopathic health care is also widespread throughout the United Kingdom. Queen Elizabeth doesn't travel unless she has her homeopathic first aid kit with her. She simply does not travel without it.

At the turn of the century, homeopathy was widely used here in the United States. There has been a decline, but it is rising again and I hope people will use it more and more. It is safe and it does, without a doubt, work.

Homeopathic remedies always heal quickly, safely, and without troublesome and dangerous side effects. They also taste good, a plus for treating children, as children are afraid of bad-tasting medicine.

I don't want to put down modern medicine. I prefer to use holistic methods for healing when I have an ailment, but the two can complement one another.

For weight loss or any health problem, I recommend that you find a good homeopathic physician and give it a try. Through homeopathy, you will discover the root problem of your weight issues. You can also contact Dr. Papon. I highly recommend that you read his book, *Homeopathy Made Simple: A Quick Reference Guide,* to help you understand exactly how it works and what to look for in a homeopathic physician.

The Most Common Causes of Weight Gain

The purposes of this book are to show you why up to now you may not have been able to lose weight for good and to show you how you can. You are going to learn how to detect what your problem is, or problems are, and how to make these new methods of losing weight with light exercise work for you.

Often overweight originates from many causes, rather than simply overeating. If you are overeating, there is a reason for it. If you are binge eating, often this is due to allergies. There can be environmental and food allergies that may be actually causing you to eat more than what you are really wanting or needing. You simply have the desire to eat and eat and then eat a little more, like you can't get that food in your mouth fast enough. Have you ever been there? More than likely this is due to allergies. A few of the other causes are hypothyroidism, *Candida albicans*, hypoglycemia, parasites, and a stressed system.

Often people get on some type of weight loss program that relies on simply lowering calories and getting into some kind of exercise regimen. These programs never work, and the weight comes right back after losing a little.

This happens for several reasons. First, you are not going to the root of the cause of your weight gain; second, most people who get on some kind of calorie-reduction, high-energy workout are not in the proper physical shape to jump into any kind of strenuous exercise program. They also may not be in the position nutritionally to start cutting calories. There is more to losing weight than simply that. I want to help you become healthy. I want to teach you what your body needs to maintain balance nutritionally and at the same time melt your body down to a new you. I want you to be comfortable in your skin and not lose out on what your body needs to maintain energy.

You will also learn how to manage stress through meditation and prayer. Positive visualization is also very important in making changes in your life, including losing weight. Believing that you can heal yourself is absolutely crucial to your success in obtaining your goal.

chapter 4

cleansing your system

Before you go and start ridding yourself of those un-wanted pounds, start with a clean system. Wouldn't it be great to not only lose the weight you want to lose, but also have a healthy body? You want to lose the weight and keep it off. I feel that it is very important to start your new life-style with a clean system. Before you improve your body with weight control, improve how your body is going to work for you. You need to regenerate new life in your body; to do this, you need to clean it up.

You are about to live life in a new way, a healthy way, have more energy, feel more comfortable in your skin, and live longer. To do this you need to clean it up before you start omitting things from your lifestyle and diet and add-ing the healthy things that will give you new life.

I want you to give your body a good housecleaning. Clean out your lower intestine and colon. Some of you reading this may be very knowledgeable about this and some of you may be hearing this for the very first time. I know when I first learned about what goes on in our intestines, my first instinct was to clean it out.

What happens is that throughout the years waste, fecal matter, builds up along the walls of your intestines and becomes a coating. You carry pounds of rot in your intestines. This rot is poison; it creates illness, decreases energy, and releases toxins into your system. Not only that, it also attracts parasites that live and grow there. A glaze of mucus builds up over the top of it, making your waste glide right through it. This damages your body by preventing it from taking in the nutrients you need and causes poor elimination. Poor eating habits, such as eating junk food, contribute to this buildup of waste and mucus. What we want to do is break this from your intestines and clean it out. Pretty gross, huh?

I've spoken to people before who have said they don't have this problem because on occasion they take a laxative. A laxative is *not* going to clean it up. It may empty you, but it is not going to clean that buildup of rot out of your body. In fact, it sometimes takes up to nine months to break this up and clean it out.

Mucus in your system, in general, is the cause of allergies, the cause of disease, the cause of pain, and the cause of death. Mucus in the body is the problem source that develops tumors, cysts, etc., bringing about old age rapidly. By old age, I'm speaking of breaking down the body to aging. Age is just a number. If you in fact take care of yourself, get all the nutrients your body needs, you can be ninety and still be young.

What we are going to do is get rid of the mucus from your entire body. It's not just a colon or intestinal thing. It's throughout your entire body.

If you clean yourself out, it will be very easy for your

body to become its normal weight, whether you are over-weight or underweight. By the way, don't say that heavy, big, or thick is normal for you. Maybe you have been a little hefty since you were a small child so that is all that you remember, but it is not what is normal for you, just what you have been living with. We are going to change that.

I remember once someone very dear to me who was overweight told me that she was quite happy with herself, being overweight was fine with her. She was happy with herself, so why should it matter to me if she felt good about herself as she was. My point was that she was not healthy. She suffered from depression; her thyroid did not work; she had *Candida*; she also had parasites and was allergic to everything under the sun. She did let me guide her. We cleaned out her system, and right away she began to lose weight. Then we went on to get rid of her parasites, killed off the yeast in her system and then we were able to get her thyroid working. The next step was for her to start working on her emotions, start loving herself. She got some therapy, found out why she was hiding behind fat, why she needed that for protection, like a blanket. Remember, it is very important to get your psychological part in balance as well as working with the physical aspect of your healing. Your body is not an independent entity. That is what this book is all about, healing yourself, not only in body, but in mind and spirit as well.

CLEANING HOUSE

A good start to your weight loss program is to clean out your colon and intestines. Remember that it can take up to nine months to complete this process. So don't wait until you have completed it before you start your program to lose the weight.

While you are doing this, I also want you to work on parasites as well. In this muck that you are carrying around you have created a wonderfully supportive feeding ground for parasites to take hold and live in.

There are different methods you can use. A few years back, I contacted The Herb Finder in St. George, Utah, to order some Turkey Rhubarb to take to cleanse myself. It did a great job, but you don't have to go out and buy Turkey Rhubarb for this purpose. This has a specific formula, but your local health food store can offer you a variety of colon formulas. Let them know exactly what it is you want to do and they will steer you in the right direction. You can also take some Slim Tea. Remember to drink a lot of water while you are doing this.

FASTING

Many experts encourage fasting as a part of purifying your body. Fasting can be very good for you and actually give you energy because you are washing out the toxins.

I don't recommend that you go on a long fast, as most of us are not in the greatest shape and it is not beneficial to you if you are indeed a mess, healthwise. Most Americans suffer from malnutrition as it is. If you feel that you want to fast, get yourself healthier first, then maybe do a fast once a month for one to four days, only if it feels right for you.

Then again, many experts feel that it is not healthy or safe to fast. Do what feels right for you, as we are all very different; do what you are attracted to doing.

THREE-DAY CLEANSING PROGRAM

Dr. John Christopher is the author of *Three-Day Cleansing Program & Mucusless Diet and Herbal Combinations.* According to Dr. Christopher, the purpose of this cleansing program is to purify the body for healing. If you are overweight, this procedure will take you down to your normal weight, and if you are underweight, it will bring you up to your normal weight. The purpose of this entire program is to eliminate mucus from the body; with the mucus out of the body, a natural healing is obtained in a more simplified way, with more convenience to the patient.

If you have any health issues, consult your physician before you begin this cleansing program.

You are not just working to lose weight—but to have a healthy body!

To begin this cleansing program, start with three days of detoxification (body purifying) therapy.

According to Dr. Christopher, supreme cleanliness is the first step toward a healthy body. Any accumulation or retention of morbid matter or waste of any kind within us will retard progress toward better health and recovery of any kind. The natural eliminative channels are the lungs, the pores of the skin, the kidneys, and the bowels.

Perspiration is the action of the sweat glands in throwing off toxins that would be injurious to us if retained in the body. The kidneys excrete the end products of food and body metabolism from the liver. Then, of course, the bowels eliminate not only the food waste but also waste matter, in the form of used-up cells and tissues. The result of our physical and mental activities, if not eliminated, causes many health problems.

This *is* going to require some work and time. You cannot fix yourself overnight. So, be patient and take one day at a time. It will be worth it. Here is your procedure:

The Detoxification Program

First thing in the morning on arising, drink 16 ounces or more of prune juice. The purpose is not just to empty the bowels, which it will do, but to draw into the intestines from every part of the body toxic matter or body waste, and eliminate it through the bowels.

During this three-day cleanse, take one or two tablespoons of olive oil three times a day, to aid in lubricating bile and liver ducts, etc.

There is quite a bit of matter that your body is going to eliminate; that matter has to be replaced, otherwise the body would be dehydrated to that extent. We are going to replace the toxic or acid material removed by drinking fruit juices. There are various types of juice therapy—apple, carrot, grape, tomato, citrus, etc.—however, you have to choose one and stick with that juice for the entire three days. Choose whichever you prefer, and literally "chew" each mouthful!

You will not eat anything all day other than your juice. By the end of the day, if you cannot take it and you are hungry, eat the fruit of whatever juice it is that you are taking. For example, if you are taking apple juice, in the evening eat an apple. If you are drinking carrot juice, in the evening eat carrots or celery. Got the picture?

Juice Therapy

General Directions (Using Apple Juice)

The apple is one of the most common fruits and is also one of the greatest herbs and blood purifiers known. There is a reason for the saying, "An apple a day keeps the doctor away." No therapeutic agents can compare with the apple tree.

Fresh apple juice is best but not always obtainable. Buy any bottled apple juice that has no preservatives or additives: pure apple juice.

After beginning with sixteen ounces of prune juice first thing in the morning, within one half-hour, take an eight-ounce glass of undiluted apple juice. Chew the juice so the saliva will mix with it. Juice must not be gulped ; drink it nice and slow. And when you do eat food, don't have drink with your meal. Chew your food thoroughly so that your saliva mixed with the food creates a liquid of its own that will trigger digestion.

Then, when desired, drink a glass of plain distilled water, followed another half-hour later with more apple juice. The general procedure is

16 ounces of prune juice first thing in the morning
8 ounces apple juice 30 minutes later
8 ounces of distilled water 30 minutes after that
Repeat the juice and distilled water each 30 minutes of the day.

Breaking up mucus during the juice cleanse generally causes constipation throughout these three days. If this is the case, take more prune juice and you will also take the Lower Bowel Formula No. 1. I'll tell you about the formula soon.

This detoxification lasts for three consecutive days. By doing this, approximately three gallons of toxic lymph will have been eliminated from your body and will have been replaced by three gallons of juices.

On the fourth and subsequent days, begin taking vegetable juices and vegetables and fruit, preferably all raw. For example, you may have some fruit for breakfast. Thirty minutes before or after you eat it, drink a glass of fruit or vegetable juice. For lunch, eat more fruit, followed by a pint of raw vegetable juice. For dinner, I recommend a salad with fresh vegetables. Then, gradually add other foods back into your diet.

Dr. Christopher says that during or after your detoxification you may feel weak. Don't be alarmed by this. Soon you will regain greater energy and vitality as a result of a cleaner and healthier body. The three-day cleanse is recommended once a month or several times a year.

Carrot Juice Therapy

The same applies to carrot juice therapy as the apple juice. The carrot juice must be used straight without diluting. Follow the same procedure as above.

Citrus Juice Therapy

This sounds great to me! A citrus combination from these juices is prepared fresh in the following proportions:

Four to six grapefruits
Two or three lemons
Enough oranges to complete a total mixture of two
    quarts.
Dilute this with two quarts of water, making one
    gallon citrus juice mixture.

Use it following the apple juice procedure.

Grape Juice Therapy

You can use unsweetened grape juice containing no additives for the three days. According to Dr. Christopher, frozen juice is not recommended because it has unacceptable additives. The best grape juice to purchase would be that from a health food store because the fruit is grown organically (no spray and organic soil). He also says that there are some regular grocery brands that have been very successful. These include Church, Tea Garden, Queen Isabell, and Welch's grape juice.

Dilute two quarts of juice with two quarts of water.
Drink eight ounces of grape juice, beginning half an hour after taking the prune juice in the morning.
Follow this with eight ounces of these diluted juices every hour thereafter until the whole four-quart mixture is finished.

Follow this procedure as you would the apple juice therapy.

Keep in mind that you do *not* dilute the apple juice or the carrot juice.

————————CONTINUED FAST————————

After the three days of juice cleanse, if you have the desire, go on to three more days using only distilled water, then a day of juice, before returning to salads and other regular foods. You don't want to eat heavy foods at once; ease into it by eating light foods and work your way gradually to heavier foods.

EXPECT A VARIETY OF RESULTS

The juice cleansing is going to make some shifts in your body. Keep in mind that you are housecleaning your entire body; it's not just your intestines and colon. There is going to be movement wherever there is mucus buildup. You may feel aches and pains, you may feel pretty icky; it will be well worth it! Keep in mind that you are going through a healing process and you must be patient.

It will take some time for a lifetime of accumulation to move on and out. Be patient. Understand that you may feel some physical reactions as you rid your body of toxins, wastes, and mucus.

Quick Reference

Supplies You Will Need

64 ounces, or 2 quarts, prune juice
9 ounces olive oil
3 gallons selected cleansing juice (apple, carrot, citrus, or grape)
3 gallons water (preferably distilled)

Cleansing Steps

Step One: Prune juice
16 oz. or more on arising in the morning
Step Two: Olive oil
One or two tablespoons three times a day
Step Three: Cleansing juice and water
8 ounces of fluid every 30 minutes,

alternating 8 ounces of juice with 8 ounces of distilled water.

Suggested Time Schedule:

7:30   16 oz. prune juice and 1–2 Tbsp. olive oil
8:00   8 oz. or more cleansing juice
8:30   8 oz, or more distilled water
9:00   8 oz. or more juice
9:30   8 oz. or more water
        Continue alternating juice and water every half-hour until noon.
Noon   8 oz. or more juice and 1–2 Tbsp. olive oil
        Continue alternating juice and water every half-hour until 5:00 p.m.
5:00 p.m.   8 oz. or more juice and 1–2 Tbsp. olive oil
        Continue alternating juice and water every half-hour until early evening
8:00 p.m.   8 oz. water every hour until retiring.

THE MUCUSLESS DIET

Dr. Christopher says that the second step to healing the body is for an individual to eliminate the mucus foods from the diet, for there is no reason to put mucus back into the body faster than you can take it out. With this preventative procedure, not only are the sinuses, the bronchi, and the lungs cleared, but the constipating mucus (catarrh) is also cleaned from the tissues of the body from the head to the bottom of the feet. The program of foods that will achieve this wonderful result is referred to as the "mucusless diet."

The Don'ts

These are mucus-forming foods:

Salt.

Eggs.

Sugar.

Meat. Eliminate all meats from the diet except a little white fish once a week, or a bit of young chicken. Try to get these that have not been fed commercial food or inoculated with formaldehyde or other antispoilage serums.

All Dairy Products. This includes milk, butter, cheese, cottage cheese, milk, yogurt, etc. You can enjoy a bland, fresh olive oil on your vegetables and salads.

Flour and Flour Products. When flour is heated and baked at high temperatures, it is changed to a mucus-forming substance. All wholesome foods are organic; where unwholesome, or dead, food is inorganic. This is the key to the whole mucusless program.

The Do's

These are supplement recommendations that will build up strength in the body and start cutting the mucus out of the tissues and remove the catarrh from the system. These are excellent revitalizing healing aids:

Cayenne. You can get this extract at the health food store or supplier. Start gradually with 1/4 teaspoon in a little cold water; drink this and follow with a glass of cold water. Add 1/4 teaspoon to this dosage every three days until you are taking one teaspoon three times a day.

Honey and Apple Cider Vinegar. Place one teaspoon of honey and one teaspoon of vinegar in warm water, so that the honey will liquefy. Sip this amount three times a day so that by the end of the day you have consumed a total of three teaspoons. Make sure that you are using raw apple cider vinegar, not distilled or other types, as these kinds are damaging to the body. The apple cider vinegar is medicinal and very beneficial. You will find more benefits of apple cider vinegar further in the book.

Kelp. If there is any indication of a thyroid problem, you should be using between five to ten kelp capsules daily; otherwise, two or more will keep the body in good condition as preventative nutrition. This can take the place of salt and will renew your thyroid gland. Kelp powder can be used on salads and other food.

Molasses. Take one tablespoon three times a day of either sorghum or blackstrap molasses.

Wheat germ oil. Take one tablespoon of a good, fresh wheat germ oil three times a day.

These things are recommended for better health. If you are overweight, you will go to your normal weight; if you are underweight, you will gain weight after you have passed your "new low," as mucus must be expelled from the body before the good flesh can be restored. For a more detailed explanation of the cleansing program and mucusless diet just described, order *Dr. Christopher's Three Day Cleansing Program, Mucusless Diet and Herbal Combinations* from Christopher Publications, P.O. Box 412, Springville, UT 84663-0777.

I highly recommend that you order Dr. Christopher's Lower Bowel Formula No. 1. It is made up of nine different herbs that help break up pounds of old, dried fecal matter that is stored in the colon, toxifying the system and keeping food from being assimilated. People tend to gorge themselves with many more times the food than they need. They are always hungry and eating, wearing out their bodies trying to get sufficient nutrition. Whereas, after the bowel is cleaned, the food is readily assimilated, and you can sustain yourself on about one-third the quantity of your current food consumption, at some four or five times more power and vitality.

Chapter 5

parasites

Part of your program in losing weight and cleaning out your system includes getting rid of any parasite that you may be carrying around so that you can start out with a nice clean body and clean organs. If you are indeed infected with parasites, it will be most difficult to lose weight, as they are one of the causes of weight gain.

Parasites are organisms that derive their food, nutrition, and shelter by living in or on other organisms. Humans may be host to more than 100 different types of parasites. It isn't something that we even like to talk about—having worms. We in the United States think that worms are found in humans only in underdeveloped countries. Wrong—they are found right here at home and have no boundaries, economic or climate-related. It is true that in some instances parasites are found more in underdeveloped countries, but we do have them here at home. You may be suffering from parasites.

I'm not even going to go into all the different types of parasites or even the most common, nor am I going to go into all the trouble that they can cause. I will give you some symptoms and how to rid yourself of these unwelcome intruders.

Parasites have to eat, so they rob us of our own nutrients. They enter our brain, heart, and lungs and make Swiss cheese of our organs. They also poison us with their toxic wastes. It can also be difficult to diagnose whether you have parasites.

An infected person may feel bloated, tired, or hungry, and have allergies, gas, unclear thinking, and generally may feel pretty toxic. Parasites like to rob us of our nutrients, taking our vitamins and amino acids. Many people become anemic and are drowsy after meals—both signs of parasites. Depression is a symptom of one particular parasite. If you are the carrier of roundworms, you may be experiencing any or all of the following:

Grinding of the teeth
Intestinal gas
Allergies
Asthma
Snoring
Digestive disturbance
Anemia
Restlessness
Weight gain around the full moon (sometimes 7–8
    pounds)
Chronic fatigue
Constipation
Diarrhea
Nervousness

HOW DO WE GET PARASITES?

Usually parasites come from unsanitary conditions where food is handled. Fruits and vegetables grown in tainted soil or not cleaned properly can be the sources of parasites. According to Hanna Kroeger, author of *Parasites: The Enemy Within*, you can get them from mountain water, undercooked beef, pork, fish, and chicken. You can also get them from your cat or dog. Rid your pets of parasites to help keep them, yourself, and your children clear of these invaders. Your pets can carry more than one kind of parasite.

RIDDING YOURSELF OF PARASITES: REMEDIES AND FOODS THAT PREVENT PARASITES

During a full moon is actually the best time to clear yourself of these unwanted guests. During the full moon is when they are most active and are multiplying. You will also gain more weight during this time because of the multiplying of the parasites. I suggest that you start your elimination of these unwanted guests five days before the full moon and on through two weeks after the full moon.

Personally, I take measures every day to keep my body clear of parasites. I might add that I have had health issues from having parasites.

You will gain weight if you have them, and besides, it's just very important to be healthy all over. If you are healthy, you will be the weight that is right for you. Meaning, you will melt down. If you are fat, you are not at a normal weight, even if that is what you have always experienced.

If you are concerned about having yourself checked out for parasites by your physician, I highly recommend it. You may want to find yourself a good homeopathic physician. He or she will treat you with natural remedies and suggest natural things for you to do rather than take drugs. What I am trying to do is to get you to let nature heal you. Drugs will make you sick, and they do kill us. Have you ever heard Dr. Joel Wallach's tapes *Dead Doctors Don't Lie?* I suggest you listen to them; you can get them at your local health food store.

There are many different things that you can take and eat to kill parasites and keep them from coming back. You may want to go to your health food store and get a parasite formula, in the homeopathy section. There are different kinds from different companies, and you may find them in a liquid form or in capsules. They are easy to take. Just put the drops under your tongue and hold them there for a minute or put the little tablets under your tongue until they dissolve for a moment. Newton puts out a formula #53 Parasite Formula that I have used; again, there are other companies that also carry a formula for this problem. The homeopathic remedies are very easy to take and quite convenient. There are other things, such as Parasite Blend by Herbs of Light, that are mixtures of different natural things that kill parasites. You put drops in water or juice and drink this several times a day. Do what you are attracted to do. Include with this different foods and herbs that will complement your remedies. You might want to consider making some of these things a part of your unending daily routine. Let's keep ourselves as healthy as we can. Not for just today, not just to lose the weight—let's stay healthy for all time.

Food and Supplements to Consider

Apple Cider Vinegar

If we are putting apple cider vinegar into our systems, worms and scavengers cannot take hold of us. I would say that that is a very important piece of information to know and practice. However, for weight loss you are going to include apple cider vinegar in your diet anyhow, in the form of the apple cider vinegar (ACV) cocktail. This is a glass of distilled water, two tablespoons of raw apple cider vinegar, and a teaspoon of honey. You may have to get raw apple cider vinegar at your health food store. I know that there is a vinegar put out by Paul and Patricia Bragg, called Bragg's Raw Apple Cider Vinegar, that can be found in many health food stores.

I remember back in 1979, I was looking to lose a couple of inches off my waist. I was going to go to a party and the dress I wanted to wear would not zip up.

I had found the dress earlier at a sale. It was beautiful; it fit like a glove and I simply had to have it. At that time I had no place to wear it—I knew that eventually an event would arise and I would have a place to wear my new dress.

Finally, a few months later, a party came up and I was ready. For the fun of it, I thought I would try on the dress. I was so proud of myself for not waiting until the last moment to find a new dress. You know how it is, you have to have a new dress for a party;

you don't want to be seen in something that everyone or someone has already seen you in. Anyhow, I decided to try it on. I could not get the zipper up. I was so upset about it that I told a neighbor. She told me what she does for a quick way of losing weight—drink the ACV cocktail every morning.

Well, I did this once a day for two weeks and measured myself once a week. I'm not big on weighing myself, but I am big on taking my measurements. If you are exercising at all, you may lose inches and not necessarily much weight. There is weight in muscle, so . . . measure yourself and keep track of your measurements.

In those two weeks, I lost two and a half inches off my waist. When I tried the dress on two days before the party, it was actually a little loose on me. I was so happy.

Even with that success, I did not know all the benefits of the ACV cocktail. For a long time, when I wanted to lose a little weight, I would start this all over again—drink the ACV cocktails, lose the weight, then stop drinking them until I needed to lose a little weight again. For some reason I had it in my mind that ACV cocktails might be too acidic for my system to be taking every day. I wish I had known then what I know now. I now drink an apple cider vinegar cocktail every day, for many reasons. It's great for losing weight, but it also takes care of and prevents many other ailments that may come along.

There is a wonderful book that I highly recommend you read to learn all about apple cider vinegar and its powerful healing ability. The Braggs will teach you in *Apple Cider Vinegar: Miracle Health System*.

I also suggest that, every once in a while, after you take a bath or shower with soap and water, moisten your skin with a little vinegar and water. Mix

1 tablespoon vinegar and 3 tablespoons water; moisten a cloth with this and go over your body after cleansing. Soap is an alkaline, and vinegar being acid gives you protection against infection and parasitic influences. It is good to keep your body slightly acidic both as a preventive measure and when treating infection. Foods that help keep the intestines acidic are apple cider vinegar and cranberry juice.

Garlic

The use of garlic goes back to ancient times as a healing remedy and as a holistic preventive medicine, and has been proven useful in the same ways today.

Garlic aids in glandular function. This will help the thyroid gland to work properly to strengthen your immune system. If your immune system is out of kilter, you can expect that disease and stress of the body and organs is going to take place, which equals weight gain.

If you suffer from *Candida albicans*, garlic will help with all your yeast-connected health problems. Some doctors and patients believe that garlic works better than the prescribed drug Nystatin. Even small amounts of garlic have beneficial effects on *Candida albicans*.

Garlic will also kill many different types of parasites. However, garlic does not kill all parasites, so I recommend that you do several things on a regular basis to keep them away.

This herb also helps stimulate and improve the body's blood purification and detoxification. We want a clean system to remain healthy and avoid any health issues. Keep in mind that this is not just a book on how to lose weight in a natural way. I want you to learn to know your body and how to detect when something is wrong with you, to be able to understand your health problems and know how to solve them. Take control and responsibility of healing yourself and keeping yourself healthy, in body, mind, and spirit.

Formula for Garlic Oil: 8 oz. of peeled or minced garlic; 4 oz. of warm extra-virgin olive oil, sufficient to cover the garlic.

There are different garlic products, such as odor-free garlic, that you can get at your health food store, and aged garlic extract (Kyolic), which Dr. William Crook highly recommends, saying he is very impressed with the reports that document the efficacy of its use.

Foods to Add to Your Diet

Apple Cider Vinegar.

Garlic.

Pumpkin Seeds. I understand that pumpkin seeds rip the skin right off the worms. You want the seeds raw and unsalted.

Papaya.

Calmyran Figs. The tiny seeds tear the skin off the worms.

Pomegranates.

Cranberry Juice.

I eat a papaya once a week. It's good to alternate among a variety of fruits, anyway. So, by eating papaya you are getting your variety of fruit and you are working on keeping yourself free of the invaders.

Some Herbs That Help Eliminate Parasites

Blue Vervain
Comfrey Leaves
Fennel Seed
Grapefruit Seed Extract
Mullein Leaves
Sage
Sesame Seed
Walnut Hulls
Wormseed
Wormwood

Dr. Christopher recommends an herbal aid for eliminating intestinal parasites. He recommends a combination of wormwood, American wormseed, tame sage, fennel, malefern, and papaya as an herbal agent for the expulsion and destruction of worms in the body. His recommended dose is to take one teaspoon each morning and night for three days. On the fourth day, drink one cup of peppermint and senna tea, using one half teaspoon of each in a cup of hot, distilled water. Pulse (rest) for two days and repeat two more times.

Foods to Avoid

Raw or undercooked beef, pork, fish, and chicken
Sugars and carbohydrates
Mountain water

Water chestnuts and watercress
Fruits or vegetables that are unwashed or washed
in questionable water

Keep in mind that your health problems, whether fatigue or just feeling lousy all over, could be because of an invasion of parasites. A diet high in carbohydrates and low in protein has been found to make parasitic infections worse. If you are having trouble with *Candida albicans* and you are having difficulty with clearing yourself of this problem, it could very well likely be due to parasites.

I recommend having yourself checked out by your physician for parasites. I would also like to see you go ahead and give yourself a good cleansing and continue to work on the prevention of parasites.

chapter 6

yeast and overweight— candida albicans

We all have yeast in our systems. If your health problems are caused by yeast, you are also having problems with your immune system. This is going to take time and a great deal of work—you didn't get this problem overnight and it's not going to go away overnight. It may take as long as a year, but the rewards of feeling good and losing the weight are indeed worth the work that it will take to do so. You are going to have to change the way you eat, and check for allergies and pollutants that aggravate the yeast in your system.

According to Dr. William G. Crook, author of *The Yeast Connection and the Woman* and *The Yeast Connection Handbook,* tests often really don't help because we all have yeast. The best way to determine if yeast is your problem is with a health history. Do you feel fatigue no matter how much rest you get, simply feel bad all over? Do you feel spacey, nervous, and forgetful? Do you suffer with digestion problems, including diarrhea, constipation, gas, or bloating? Are there reproductive problems, including more than normal menstrual cramping, menstrual irregularities, and premenstrual tensions?

Candida fungi live in everyone's bodies, including yours. They live in mucous membranes, in the digestive tract and in the vagina. You may not be bothered by digestive symptoms or vaginitis. However, if you have the symptoms I have named, I would safely assume that you do have *Candida*.

Can men have *Candida*? Absolutely! This is not a female problem; men and women alike suffer from it. Men may feel grumpy, irritable, have "jock itch," athlete's foot, and prostate problems.

What is needed here is to discourage the growth of *Candida*. To do this we have to eliminate the foods that feed this yeast—go on a diet that will discourage its growth especially in the digestive tract and vagina.

Many medical disorders are indeed related to yeast yet often not acknowledged by the medical profession. Yeast weakens the immune system, possible resulting in headaches, fatigue, and depression. You may also have multiple sclerosis, psoriasis, cancer, or develop AIDS. You will be more susceptible to infections and allergies.

According to Dr. Crook, you can suspect *Candida* of playing a role in your health if any of the following are true for you.

> You have taken antibiotics for acne.
> You have had prolonged or repeated courses of antibiotics for sinusitis, bronchitis, urinary tract or ear infections.
> You have taken birth control pills or have been pregnant.
> Your symptoms are aggravated by tobacco smoke, perfumes, auto fumes, and other chemical odors.

You feel lethargic, drained, or depressed.

You have nervous system symptoms such as poor memory, the inability to concentrate, headaches, or feeling spaced out or irritable.

You have muscle weakness.

Incoordination is a problem—you bump into things while you are walking.

You are troubled by vaginal yeast infections or other disorders involving the sex organs or urinary system.

You have athlete's foot, jock itch, and other skin infections.

Heartburn, bloating, abdominal pain, gas, constipation, or diarrhea occur.

There is pain or swelling of your joints.

You have frequent coughs, sore throats, or nasal problems.

You just feel "icky."

Your symptoms flare up on damp days or in moldy places or when you eat or drink foods that promote yeast growth.

You are going to have to go on a very strict diet to control your problems and rid yourself of the foods that make this yeast grow. You will remove sugar from your diet. You will remove anything and everything that promotes the growth of yeast. So, you will stop eating sweets, foods that contain yeast, wheat, mushrooms, vinegar, beer, and wine. You will also need to remove processed and packaged foods from your diet. (You know—just-add-hamburger meals and boxed macaroni and cheese—those kinds of foods.) Also remove foods such as white flour that contain sugar or turn into sugar after you eat them.

You are going to have to start living differently from the past. You will have to break old habits and build new healthy ones. Is cutting sugar out of your diet difficult? At first it may be a tough order, but when you sit down and weigh the results of how you will feel in comparison with how you feel today, believe me the changes will be well worth it. Basically, knock out *junk* foods. In Suzanne Somers' *Eat Great, Lose Weight,* she calls junk foods, *funky* foods. *Funky* or *junky,* lose them!

So many of you want to wave a magic wand and make the fat disappear. It is not that easy, but all good things in life are worth the work that is involved to manifest them. The thing to remember here is that when we get everything in your system balanced, you will feel so good, have so much energy, deter disease, have more passion for life, be at optimal good health, and feel comfortable in your skin. You will live a whole lot longer and stay young. I've mentioned this young thing quite a bit. I don't know about you, but I want to feel and look young. While I have no problem with the thought of getting older, I don't feel that we have to hurry it along—you are as young as you feel and you become what you believe you are. If you believe that you are an old lady, an old man, you will be just that. Be careful with your verbiage, there is great energy in words and in the thought; you truly do become what you believe you are.

It seems that I have had bouts with yeast off and on for what seems like forever. One of my problems was that I would work on ridding myself of the *Candida,* staying on the diet, but not staying on it quite long enough. I would lose the weight, get the yeast under some control, get my thyroid working, and then bang! boom! the weight would creep back on and my thyroid would fail to work, and the padding would grow back onto my body. I wasn't staying on the diet quite long enough. (Long enough meaning maybe a year or two.) I would go on the diet for a few months and think that that would cover the situation. I would be feeling great, so everything must be working. Well, sometimes it takes a year or two to rid your body of the yeast; the real trick is to stay on the diet. Keep sugar out of your system and be healthy for the rest of your life. It's okay to splurge occasionally and eat whatever you feel like eating; don't feel bad or guilty about it. Simply once in a while—splurge!

However, I have found that I really don't want sugar and if I have it, I feel lousy the next day. You'll also find that removing allergens will improve how you feel, helping you lose weight. I will show you later in the book how to test yourself for allergies. The other day, I thought I wanted a chocolate bar. I really didn't want it; it just sounded good to me. I went out and bought two of them. I ate part of one and felt nauseous, had to stop and throw the rest of it away along with the unopened candy bar. The next day I felt very bad physically. I am allergic to chocolate, and not having had any for such a long time, it hit me like a ton of bricks. There was a time when I felt that I had to eat chocolate on a daily basis. I was addicted to it; it also fed my *Candida*. You and your body will crave what you are allergic to, rather the yeast in your system will crave sugar; the yeast has to be fed or it will go away. Yeast wants to grow and grow, colonize wherever it can.

Most people think that for women if you have yeast, it must be a vaginal thing. I have had problems with yeast, but it has been about twenty years since I have had vaginal yeast. I have had yeast in my intestines and in my lungs. So, don't think that just because you don't have a vaginal yeast infection, you don't have any yeast in your system. If you are a man, you too are prone to having yeast. We all are; it's a matter of having good or bad yeast in our system.

Children, and even babies, can have problems with *Candida*. If you are a man, you too will follow the same directions given in this book. I don't want you all to think that I am leaning only toward women's issues, although there are more women with *Candida albicans* than there are men that suffer from this problem. Many illnesses are connected to yeast.

I have included Dr. Crook's questionnaire and score sheet in this chapter, which should help you evaluate the possibility of yeast being a problem in your inability to lose weight. When we take care of your yeast problems, we will also take care of your immune system. When you have yeast in your system, your immune system is very low, which makes you susceptible to diseases.

You should find a physician to help you with this, if you can find someone that leans toward holistic ways of healing, or is at least open to your natural ways of healing yourself without drugs. There are many in the medical field that may disagree with the yeast findings because often yeast cannot be proven. Often a physician will prescribe Nystatin or Diflucan to aid in ridding you of yeast. Dr. Crook prescribes these medications, along with urging you to do other natural treatments as well. These drugs simply speed the recovery from yeast problems. These are antifungal drugs that kill yeast and yeastlike fungi.

In 1997, I went to Europe and spent a couple of months there. When I left the States, I was very healthy. No signs of *Candida*, no parasites, and my thyroid was working properly. One of my sisters lives in Sweden, where I spent a month with her through the holidays. The visit was great. However, I came home unbelievably ill. For one, I picked up a parasite, or three! I came home with yeast growing rampant throughout my body. How did this happen?

I have allergies to dust and different molds, not to mention different foods. My sister has a business making jams and jellies that have become quite famous throughout Europe. When she puts her jams and jellies in jars, there are some jar lids that don't seal properly. These jars cannot be sold and are no good unless they are going to be eaten at that time. There is only so much room in the refrigerator and stomach for so much jam. Which by the way, I do not indulge in, it's *all* sugar. She took the lids off the bad jars and had them sitting in flats. As you can imagine, mold grew on the top of the products, and this mold permeated the house. After a couple of weeks, I felt very poorly and suggested that we clean it all up, but every time I went down to the cellar I could hardly breathe. I went down there quite a bit as we took turns adding wood to the furnace, which was down in the cellar. This caused yeast to grow throughout my body.

Yeast doesn't always happen because of the foods you eat. It is often the things in your environment such as tobacco smoke, perfumes, diesel fumes, and other chemical odors that aggravate yeast.

The good old mold that you find in the bathtub can be a problem for you. It will be helpful to keep your environment clean, keeping molds and dust under control. Then again, some cleaning products can also affect this problem. Sound like it's never ending? It can be ended and I will help to guide you through this.

It is also very important to read as much as you can about health in general and ways of improving it. There are always findings about ways of bettering your health, new findings regarding a simple mineral or vitamin that can make a world of difference in how you live. In the back of the book, I will have some information on how you can find out more about yeast-related problems.

It is very important to work with your physician. Get a physical exam; you want to make sure that your symptoms are not caused by some other disorder. Although it is difficult to diagnose *Candida albicans*, a great deal of the diagnosis is going to be determined on case history. However, if you just feel lousy all over and have yeast-related symptoms, my guess would be that yeast is your problem.

I would simply take things into my own hands and go on the strict diet, and include everything that is recommended that complements the diet. Remember that no two people are alike and that what may work for one person may not work for another. Each case is individual and needs to be treated as such.

CANDIDA QUESTIONNAIRE

AND SCORE SHEET

Dr. Crook has generously allowed me to use his questionnaire and score sheet for my book. It is designed for adult women and men only, and is not appropriate to be used by children.

The questions in Section A focus on factors in your medical history that promote the growth of *Candida albicans,* along with items in the history that are often found in people with yeast-related problems.

In Section B, you'll find a list of 23 symptoms often present in patients with yeast-related health problems. Section C consists of 33 other symptoms that are sometimes seen in people with yeast-related problems—yet they may also be found in people with other disorders.

According to Dr. Crook, filling out and scoring this

questionnaire should help you and your physician evaluate the possibility of your health problems being related to *Candida albicans.* However, it will not provide you with an automatic answer.

Section A: History*

Record point value shown for every yes answer pertaining to your health history.

Point Score

1. Have you taken tetracyclines or other antibiotics for acne for one month (or longer)? (35)

   _____

2. Have you at any time in your life taken broad-spectrum antibiotics or other antibacterial medication for respiratory, urinary, or other infections for two months or longer, or in shorter courses four or more times in a one-year period? (35)

   _____

3. Have you taken a broad-spectrum antibiotic drug— even in a single dose? (6)

   _____

4. Have you, at any time in your life, been bothered by persistent prostatis, vaginitis, or other problems affecting your reproductive organs? (25)

   _____

---

*   The *Candida* questionnaire and score sheet is reproduced in full from *The Yeast Connection Handbook* by William G. Crook, M.D., Professional Books, Inc., P.O. Box 3494, Jackson, TN 38301. Used with permission.

5. Are you bothered by memory or concentration problems? Do you sometimes feel spaced out? (20)

_____

6. Do you feel "sick all over" yet, in spite of visits to many different physicians, the causes haven't been found? (20)

_____

7. Have you been pregnant . . .

two or more times? (5)

_____

one time? (3)

_____

8. Have you taken birth control pills . . .

For more than two years? (15)

_____

For six months to two years? (8)

_____

9. Have you taken steroids orally, by injection, or by inhalation . . .

For more than two weeks? (15)

_____

For two weeks or less? (6)

_____

10. Does exposure to perfumes, insecticides, fabric shop odors, and other chemicals provoke . . .

Moderate to severe symptoms? (20)

_____

Mild symptoms? (5)

_____

11. Does tobacco smoke really bother you? (10)

_____

12. Are your symptoms worse on damp, muggy days or in moldy places? (20)

_____

13. Have you had athlete's foot, ringworm, "jock itch," or other chronic fungous infections of the skin or nails? Have such infections been . . .

Severe or persistent? (20)

_____

Mild to moderate? (10)

_____

14. Do you crave sugar? (10)

_____

Total Score, Section A: _____

Section B: Major Symptoms

For each of your symptoms, enter the appropriate figure in the Point Score column:

If a symptom is occasional or mild (3)
If a symptom is frequent and/or moderately severe (6)
If a symptom is severe and/or disabling (9)

Add total score and record it at the end of this section.

Point Score

1. Fatigue or lethargy

_____

2. Feeling of being "drained"

_____

3. Depression or manic depression

_____

4. Numbness, burning, or tingling

_____

5. Headache

_____

6. Muscle aches

_____

7. Muscle weakness or paralysis

_____

8. Pain and/or swelling in joints

_____

9. Abdominal pain

_____

10. Constipation and/or diarrhea

_____

11. Bloating, belching, or intestinal gas

_____

12. Troublesome vaginal burning, itching, or discharge

_____

13. Prostatis

_____

14. Impotence

_____

15. Loss of sexual desire or feeling

_____

16. Endometriosis or infertility

_____

17. Cramps and/or other menstrual irregularities

_____

18. Premenstrual tension

_____

19. Attacks of anxiety or crying

_____

20. Cold hands or feet, low body temperature

_____

21. Hypothyroidism

_____

22. Shaking or irritable when hungry

_____

23. Cystitis or interstitial cystitis

_____

Total Score, Section B   _____

Section C: Other Symptoms

For each of your symptoms, enter the appropriate figure in the Point Score column:

If a symptom is occasional or mild (1)
If a symptom is frequent and/or moderately severe (2)
If a symptom is severe and/or disabling (3)

Add total score and record it at the end of this section.

Point Score

1. Drowsiness, including inappropriate drowsiness

_____

2. Irritability

_____

3. Incoordination

_____

4. Frequent mood swings

_____

5. Insomnia

_____

6. Dizziness/loss of balance

_____

7. Pressure above ears . . .feeling of head swelling

_____

8. Sinus problems . . .tenderness of cheekbones or forehead

_____

9. Tendency to bruise easily

_____

10. Eczema, itching eyes

_____

11. Psoriasis

_____

12. Chronic hives (urticaria)

_____

13. Indigestion or heartburn

_____

14. Sensitivity to milk, wheat, corn, or other common foods

_____

15. Mucus in stools

_____

16. Rectal itching

_____

17. Dry mouth or throat

_____

18. Mouth rashes, including "white" tongue

_____

19. Bad breath

_____

20. Foot, hair, or body odor not relieved by washing

_____

21. Nasal congestion or postnasal drip

_____

22. Nasal itching

_____

23. Sore throat

_____

24. Laryngitis, loss of voice

_____

25. Cough or recurrent bronchitis

_____

26. Pain or tightness in chest

_____

27. Wheezing or shortness of breath

_____

28. Urinary frequency or urgency

_____

29. Burning on urination

_____

30. Spots in front of eyes or erratic vision

_____

31. Burning or tearing eyes

_____

32. Recurrent infections or fluid in ears

_____

33. Ear pain or deafness

_____

Total Score, Section A   _____

Total Score, Section B   _____

Total Score, Section C   _____

Grand Total Score   _____

The Grand Total Score will help you and your physician decide if your health problems are yeast connected. Scores in women will run higher, as seven items in the questionnaire apply exclusively to women, while only two apply exclusively to men.

Yeast-connected health problems are almost certainly present in women with scores over 180, and in men with scores over 140.

Yeast-connected health problems are probably present in women with scores over 120, and in men with scores over 90.

Yeast-connected health problems are possibly present in women with score over 60, and in men with scores over 40.

With scores of less than 60 in women and 40 in men, yeast is less apt to cause health problems.

When you go to the doctor, if you are seeing a general physician, make sure that he or she is educated in yeast problems. If your doctor wants to do any skin tests to see if *Candida* is the problem, don't do it. From what I understand, often doctors will want to do this test, which actually tells them nothing about having *Candida*. It makes for very expensive testing that is not necessary and will cost you a pretty penny.

I would like to see people take their health responsibilities into their own hands. Your body can heal itself if you are practicing preventive medicine. When you eat healthy foods, take supplements, and learn your body—learn as much as you can about natural healing—you can avoid illness. I'm all for longevity, feeling high in energy, and simply being as healthy as I possibly can. Keep in mind that sugar makes yeast multiply!

You need to put yourself on the *Candida albicans* diet. If you think this is your problem but are not sure, go on the diet. You have nothing to lose; you will be healthier whether yeast is your problem or not; and you will lose weight. If you do have yeast problems and you go on the diet to kill off the yeast you can lose the weight and keep it off with no "yo-yoing!"

YOUR DIET TO RID YOURSELF OF *CANDIDA ALBICANS*

First, pick a convenient time to start this diet; you don't want to start right before the holidays or right before you go on vacation or go to visit someone. Decide when you are going to do this and take it seriously. The results will be well worth it.

According to Dr. Crook, the first thing you should do is clean out your kitchen. Get rid of the sugar, corn syrup, white bread and other flour products, soft drinks, and most ready-to-eat cereals. (Cookies, cakes, chocolate, ketchup, ice-cream, cola—you've got the picture.) Replace these foods with more vegetables, including some that you do not ordinarily eat. Rid your kitchen of foods containing hydrogenated and partially hydrogenated oils, replacing them with unrefined oils such as flaxseed, canola, and olive oil.

Avoid yeasty foods and beverages, especially dried fruits, mushrooms, condiments, alcohol, juices except freshly squeezed juices, leavened breads, bagels, pastries, pretzels, pizza, and rolls.

After two or three weeks of being on the diet, and your health has improved, Crook suggests that you try a yeast food and see if it bothers you.

He also reminds us that diets are not forever and that after a month or so, you will be able to relax a bit.

I know I have said all of this before, but now we are beginning our diet.

Chemical Exposures

People with yeast-related problems are almost always sensitive to chemicals they encounter on a daily basis. Some of these are tobacco smoke, perfumes, colognes, glues, carpet odors, paints, formaldehyde, insecticides, diesel fumes, and other traffic odors.

Many of these things are impossible to avoid. However, you can clear your home of some of these irritants. Start by getting rid of odorous bathroom and kitchen chemicals, insecticides, and other inhalants. After you do this, your symptoms should begin to disappear.

You may react to chemicals in and on your food. So where possible, eat organic foods and choose prepared foods in glass containers.

Clean Your Fruits and Vegetables

When I get home from the grocery store, I fill my sink with about a gallon of water, add a capful of bleach to it, and soak the nuts and vegetables I have just purchased for twenty minutes. I then run cold water to rinse them for another twenty minutes. This will clean them up dramatically.

Change Your Lifestyle

Get plenty of fresh air, sunshine, exercise, and the sleep you need. Stop lying around the house; get up and move, walk, have some fun.

Psychological Support

To strengthen your immune system and overcome your health problems, Dr. Crook says that besides the obvious diet changes, you also need to get some emotional and psychological help, which includes encouragement, love, touch, hugs, and laughing.

Nutritional Supplements

Vitamins, minerals, and other supplements are of great importance, especially for people with yeast-related health problems. Here is a list of some of the things that you need to add to your new lifestyle:

Multivitamin, mineral, and antioxidant preparations. These should be yeast-free, sugar-free, and color-free. I personally take a liquid supplement called Total Toddy, distributed by Soaring Eagle. I'm not going to go into exactly what is in it—go into your local health food store and check it out. It has just about everything in the mineral and vitamin family that you could possibly need.

Essential fatty acids (EFAs). These include flaxseed oil, which is the richest known source of omega-3 fatty acids. They also contain other oils, including omega-6 EFAs. The usual dose is one or two tablespoons a day, you can take it straight or grind flax seeds to make a powder.

Oils that are rich in omega-6 EFAs include evening primrose oil, borage, and black currant seed oils. These oils are especially recommended for women with PMS and certain types of eczema. Evening primrose oil will also help you to curb your appetite.

Nonprescription Anti-Candida Substances

After you have done all the above, you are ready to take substances which help control *Candida* overgrowth in your intestinal tract and restore normal bacteria.

Probiotics. These are preparations of lactobacillus acidophilus and other probiotic bacteria that help crowd out *Candida* in your digestive tract. Brand names include Vitalplex, Prime-Plex, Vital-Dophilus, Kyo-Dophilus, Kala, BifidoBiotics and Lactibacillus sporogenes, Geneflora, Maxidophilus, Acidophilus DDSI, Flora Balance, GI Flora, Primadophilus, Saccaromyces boulardi, and Superdophilus. The usual dose is one-quarter to one-half teaspoon of powder or 1 to 2 capsules, 1 to 4 times a day.

I take Jarro-Dophilus+FOS, plus Nutra Flora, by Jarroe Formulas. This is taken as follows: one-fourth teaspoon per day with unchilled water twenty to sixty minutes after eating.

Citrus seed extracts. These are available in capsules and liquids. The usual dose is 1 or 2 capsules or 2 to 6 drops of liquid, 1 to 3 times a day. The liquid must be diluted in at least 4 oz. of water and stirred well. According to Dr. Crook, these extracts are as effective as Nystatin and caprylic acid in treating patients with yeast overgrowth in the intestinal tract. They are also useful in treating patients with giardiasis and other intestinal parasites. I highly recommend that you *do* take this.

Garlic cloves and/or Kyolic tablets, capsules, or drops.

Caprylic acid. Brand names include Mycopryl 400 or 680, Capricin, Caprystatin and Kaprycidin A. The usual dose is 1 to 2 capsules with each meal.

Mathtake (Teriminalia catappa). An herbal product that was just introduced in the United States in the mid-1980s by Michael Weiner, Ph.D., Mathtake is a very affordable, easy-to-use medicine. It doesn't taste bad, is portable, and does not require refrigeration. You simply add a tea bag of the Mathtake to a cup of boiling water. Dr. Crook prescribes it first in treating children and adults with mild to moderate *Candida*-related health problems.

Yogurt. Don't forget that you can also eat plain yogurt. I personally can't stand it, but I eat it because

I know that it is good for me. (I sprinkle cinnamon on it to add a better flavor.)

Pau d'Arco (La Pacho or taheebo). This comes in many forms, including as a tea. I recommend you go to your health food store and ask questions about it. I take Yeast Releaf, Pau D'Arco—Black Walnut Complex, by Herbs ETC. taking 10–25 drops 4 times a day in a cup of water. It comes in a 1 fluid ounce bottle with a dropper.

Oil of Oregano.

Oregano. Take 1 to 3 drops in a glass of distilled water, once a day.

There are also different prescribed medications that your physician can give you that are safe to take.

Food Allergies and Sensitivities

During the diagnostic part of your diet, avoid fruits because many of them turn into sugar once they are in your intestinal tract.

After the first two or three weeks of your diet, do a fruit challenge:

Take a bite of a small banana. Ten minutes later, eat a second bite. If there is no reaction in the next hour, eat the whole banana.

If you do not develop any symptoms after eating the banana, repeat the challenge, one fruit at a time, in following days.

If you show no symptoms after eating these fruits, we can safely say that you can eat fruits in moderation, but take it easy with them.

Note: If you find you can add fruits to your diet, be sure to choose from a variety, as you will with other foods.

Following the Diet

It will be difficult at first to be on this diet. The first few days will be the worse. You may feel pretty irritable or even feel angry at everyone and everything. This is because your body will be craving the foods you are avoiding, especially sugar. After about three weeks, when your symptoms improve, do a challenge, as described above, on the foods you have been avoiding. After you try one of the foods, wait another twenty-four to forty-eight hours before you try another food.

It can take a few minutes, or it can take hours, before you feel the symptoms. Possible symptoms are headache, stuffy nose, itching, coughing, or urinary frequency.

If you don't feel any symptoms, try the same food the next day.

Keep a diary of what goes on with your body when you eat these foods. You'll find that any time you avoid a food allergen for five to seven days, you will get the allergic symptoms almost immediately after eating it. If you avoid the food for three weeks or more, you may have to eat the food two or three days in a row before you develop any symptoms.

Keep in mind that if you show a reaction to a food, you will also react to any food from that food family. When you come across a food that gives you a reaction, eliminate that food indefinitely. If you get a reaction to milk, you will probably get a reaction to beef as well. Get the connection?

Chicken and eggs are the same! I don't want this to sound too complex; I simply want you to be able to test yourself for food allergies. It's actually much easier than you think. Keep a log of what you try. Don't worry about starving; there are plenty of healthy foods out there for you to eat.

When you are trying different foods, eat them in their purest form. For example, eat an egg soft- or hard-boiled. Drink whole milk. For citrus, eat an orange or drink fresh-squeezed orange juice; don't use frozen or canned. Use Baker's cooking chocolate or Hershey's cocoa powder. Eat the powder with a spoon or add it to a little water to make a drink. Eat corn on the cob, pure corn syrup, grits, or hominy. Do the same with sugar: eat a lump of sugar or add a little to some water and drink it. Keep in mind that we are looking for a reaction, not necessarily for a way to continue eating sugar.

This is just a test to see what may be causing you to feel poorly. For example, if you do have a reaction to eggs, you may find that you can eat chicken in moderation. This is all a trial-and-error test.

By eliminating all the foods that feed the *Candida* and adding different alternative health treatments, you will clean up your body, lose weight, and rid yourself of different chronic health disorders. Your immune system will improve; if you are suffering physically, watch this disappear as well.

chapter 7

hypothyroidism

A low thyroid function may be affecting your weight, your body, your emotions, and other aspects of your existence.

I remember that when I was pregnant with my first daughter in 1969, I was very ill. My doctor told me that my thyroid was overactive. I really had no idea what that meant. I don't recall even asking him any questions about it.

That was a time, I think, when most people went to the doctor and simply accepted what the doc said, took what the doctor ordered, and didn't really ask a lot of questions. I don't recall my doctor checking my thyroid ever again.

I had over a period of time two more daughters. I also had six miscarriages, which the doctor said were caused by my negative Rh factor. I accepted that, but today I often wonder if my thyroid's imbalance could have played a part. It's very common to miscarry easily when your thyroid is not working properly.

I went through years marked by some very serious health issues. Depression was one of them. There were times when I seemed to be fine and other times when I had such serious depression that I thought I was truly crazy or on my way there. I also suffered from PMS. I found out much later that this was all brought on by hypothyroidism.

A few years ago, Dr. Don Papon ran some tests and found many things wrong with me. Included in the list was my thyroid. Further tests showed my thyroid was not working because of *Candida albicans*. To get my thyroid working, we had to kill off the yeast. So, I had to control the yeast to get the thyroid working. Of course, the best method of kick-starting your thyroid is increasing your intake of iodine. However, you don't just start working on getting the thyroid working correctly; you have to go to the root of the problem and fix whatever has thrown it off. Many people out there on thyroid medication lose a little weight. However, even with the medication, they still have to go to the cause or the weight will come back.

Throughout the years there have been different methods designed to test the thyroid, with many failing attempts. The British were first to recognize thyroid deficiency, and the first to compare various thyroid diagnostic tests. Dr. Broda Barnes developed the Basal Temperature Test, which is very accurate. You can perform it yourself with a common oral thermometer. This test is practiced worldwide by physicians in preference to blood tests, which are specific for hypothyroidism but not sensitive enough.

BASAL TEMPERATURE TEST

A man can take the test on any day, but it's a different story for women. A woman's temperature fluctuates during her menstrual cycle. It is at its lowest during ovulation and highest shortly before the start of her menstrual flow. If you are a woman in menstrual years, it is best to measure your basal temperature during the second and third days after flow starts. You can take your temperature on any day if your physical stage falls before the menarche or after menopause.

Taking the Test

Before going to bed, take an oral thermometer with you, shake it down well, and place it on your nightstand. When you wake up in the morning, place it snugly in your armpit. Keep it there for exactly ten minutes. Watch the clock; it is very important that it remain there for the full ten minutes. Be sure to take your temperature as soon as you wake up, before you do anything; don't even get up to go to the bathroom until you have taken your temperature. The normal range is 97.8° to 98.2°. A reading below this strongly suggests low thyroid function. If your temperature is above the normal range, you're more than likely to have an overactive thyroid gland or possibly an infection.

COMMON HYPOTHYROIDISM SYMPTOMS

Unfortunately, the thyroid is one of the most obvious causes of so many illnesses, yet gets the least attention paid to it by mainstream medicine. The thyroid gland is one of the body's master glands, with hypothyroidism a common, unsuspected cause of major illness and, often, obesity or weight gain.

According to Stephen Langer, M.D., and James F. Scheer, who wrote *Solved: The Riddle of Weight Loss*, this is the list of the most common symptoms of hypothyroidism, in the order of their most common frequency:

Fatigue
Feeling cold, particularly in the hands and feet
Weight gain or inability to lose weight, despite constant attempts at dieting
Lethargy
Dry, coarse skin
Swelling eyelids
Coarse hair
Pale skin
Enlarged heart
Faulty memory
Constipation
Hair loss
Difficult breathing
Swelling feet
Hoarseness
Nervousness
Depression
Menstrual problems
Loss of sexual desire and enjoyment of sex
Impotence
Heart palpitation.
Emotional instability
Brittle nails
Muscle weakness, pain
Pain in joints
Poor concentration and memory
Anemia
Atherosclerosis
High cholesterol levels

According to Langer and Scheer, if you have two of the first five symptoms and six or more of the latter, you're more than likely hypothyroid. A good question to ask yourself is whether you or anyone in your family ever had a goiter. A goiter is brought on by lack of iodine; lack of iodine creates hypothyroidism.

Dr. Broda Barnes, author of *Hypothyroidism: The Unsuspected Illness,* and the ultimate know-it-all of the thyroid gland, says the thyroid is the main cause for illnesses including lupus; miscarriages, often multiple miscarriages like myself with six; eczema; arthritis; and many others. Then, of course, there is weight gain. This book is about more than weight; I also want you to watch your entire health. There is more to losing weight than dieting, and exercise; we also need to be healthy on all levels.

Still another common affliction involving the thyroid, according to Dr. Steven Langer, is Hashimoto's thyroiditis or autoimmune thyroiditis (AIT). This condition can block serious weight campaigns. Langer says that in different stages of this serious illness, a person can manifest symptoms of hypothyroidism or hyperthyroidism. The most common symptoms of thyroiditis are

Profound fatigue
Memory loss
Depression
Nervousness
Allergies
Heartbeat irregularity
Muscle and joint pain
Sleep disturbances
Reduced sex drive
Menstrual problems
Suicidal tendencies

Digestive disorders
Headaches and ear pain
Lump in the throat
Problems swallowing

Deep fatigue and psychological problems seem to be the most prevalent of complaints of AIT. Often there is nervousness, and maybe even panic attacks, that need psychological attention. It has been very common for people with AIT (95% of whom are female) to actually commit themselves into a psychiatric ward because of how they are feeling. They often are put on drugs such as lithium, only making their condition worsen. Also, often what they do to make themselves feel better is to eat, which only makes the depression worse.

If you feel in fact that you may be suffering from AIT, I recommend that you have your physician do a thorough test for this ailment. I personally would go to a homeopathic physician because I know that he or she would treat me with natural products and there would be no attempt to put me on any kind of drug. I recommend a doctor that is nutritionally oriented. For additional information, read Dr. Barnes's book. Learn as much as you can about your body and your health. Take what works for you. Try different things until you get your system balanced.

MAKE YOUR THYROID PERFORM

There are two ways to make your thyroid gland function normally. One is making changes or additions to your diet; the other is taking natural, desiccated thyroid prescribed by your physician. For supplements, choose kelp and cod liver oil. (Don't freak out, you can now go to the health food store and get different flavors of cod liver oil.) You can almost always correct your condition by simply adding more iodine-containing foods to your diet. Many foods have high amounts of iodine in them. There is iodine in salt. However, you don't want to increase your salt intake because it can create new problems, such as weight gain and high blood pressure.

If you are a vegetarian, you may be doing yourself some harm unless you truly understand nutrition. You may be eliminating some vital sources of different vitamins and minerals that make your thyroid gland perform. For example, it is believed that the lack of vitamin A reduces thyroid hormone secretion. You also need to make sure that you are getting sufficient amounts of the B vitamins; if you are deficient in these, the thyroid gland is not going to produce hormones your body needs and it will be handicapped in its job of converting the iodine into thyroid hormones.

Good food sources of vitamin B_2 are beef liver, beef heart, nonfat dry milk, and almonds; the richest of all is brewer's yeast. Your thyroid gland also needs the vitamin B_6, provided by leg of veal, fresh fish, beef liver, kidney, avocado, bananas, walnuts, prunes, and wheat germ. B_{12}, which is found mainly in animal products, is also needed.

The lack of vitamin C can actually make your thyroid gland bleed. So, as you see, it is very important to take good care of yourself all the way around to have your thyroid gland working properly. Lack of these vitamins will also affect other areas of your well-being. Let's get healthy. The results will be energy and longevity. Life is filled with deliciousness. Let's be around as long as we can, feeling good and keeping the wonderful feeling of youthfulness.

There are other causes for your thyroid to stop functioning properly besides the lack of iron and certain vitamins. Some of these are antibiotics, prednisone, and estrogen; thyocyanide in cigarette smoke and fluoride in drinking water also hinder the thyroid gland from working.

I only drink spring, distilled, and seltzer water and always put about a quarter of a lemon in it. You should be drinking at least eight glasses of water a day. I buy large jugs of spring water and go through a gallon of water about every two days. I don't believe you can drink too much water. I want to make sure that I get as much citrus as I can. I don't have the lemon just for my thyroid; I have it for better health and well-being. Once you make the changes in your lifestyle, you won't want to do things any differently.

Although the best sources of iodine are kelp and cod liver oil, you can also get iodine in your diet through seafood, especially shrimp. I love shrimp, and what a wonderful excuse to have to eat it often—I need my iodine. Lobster and crab also carry iodine as well as saltwater fish such as halibut, cod, herring, and haddock. Now don't go crazy taking in as much iodine as you possibly can; too much of anything is not good. Most of the time low thyroid can be corrected through your diet. For a more serious condition, change your diet and go to a physician who is nutritionally oriented or a preventive-medicine specialist. Dr. Langer prescribes Armour and says to make sure that your doctor knows about the Barnes Basal Temperature test. There is also raw glandular thyroid that is sold in nutritional centers. According to Langer, the best and safest form of iodine supplement is kelp tablets. I live in Norfolk, Virginia, and fortunately only twenty minutes from me, in

Virginia Beach, is the Heritage Store, which I believe is the second largest health food and New Age store in the country. They make a product that I highly recommend—Sea-Adine, which is made by this store for this store only. I take it as a source of iodine; it is made from dulse, a type of seaweed. Sea-Adine is recommended in the Edgar Cayce readings.

I send many people to the Heritage Store to get this product, and after following my advice, they are having wonderful results with their thyroids and are melting down to the weight that they have either been or have always wanted to be—and are keeping their weight off.

chapter 8

carnitine— the fat burner and energizer

What is carnitine? Carnitine is a compound, produced in small amounts by our bodies, that turns fat into energy. In that way, it is similar to the B vitamins.

According to Robert Crayhon, author of *The Carnitine Miracle*, and one of the top ten nutritionists in the United States, carnitine works like a forklift, picking up fats and dropping them off where the body will burn them. Carnitine carries fat and puts it into the part of the cell that burns the fat. We like this!

Carnitine will also improve your all-around well-being. We age and get disease because our cells die; they run out of energy. Carnitine solves this problem. What you want to know about right now is how to lose weight. With carnitine, you will lose weight; you will also improve many other aspects of your life. It's given to people with heart trouble, diabetes, hypoglycemia, and many other ailments.

A lot of athletes take carnitine. It gives them more energy and greater endurance. It helps considerably for sex. Why? More endurance, more energy, and more stamina = better sex! (Robert Erdmann, Ph.D., in his book *The Amino Revolution*, calls carnitine the "Don Juan" amino for this very reason.)

While carnitine is completely safe to take, it is not recommended for someone with serious problems with depression. Check with your doctor first. However, we often can become mildly depressed because we sit and dwell on our problems. Carnitine will give you energy; you aren't going to want to be sitting around; you will want to be productive. I find it better than evening primrose oil, although I recommend evening primrose oil to help with food cravings. Did I mention that carnitine melts cellulite?

WHICH FOODS CONTAIN CARNITINE?

Carnitine is found predominantly in meat and animal products. Red meat is the best source; mutton and lamb have the highest levels of carnitine. Chicken and turkey also contain carnitine, but not as much as red meats. Carnitine is also found in a lesser degree in milk and dairy products. If you are lacking other nutrients, the ones that help in retrieving the carnitine from these foods, you have to take the supplement carnitine. If you seriously want to lose weight, you take carnitine! There isn't enough carnitine in the foods that contain it to really help you transfer fat into energy. If you are a vegetarian, you are probably not getting any carnitine into your system.

HOW MUCH CARNITINE SHOULD I TAKE?

Most of us consume about 50 mg of carnitine per day in our diet. Those who eat large quantities of red meats get more. There is evidence that for optimal health you should be getting at least 250 to 500 mg daily. The problem with carnitine is that people don't take enough. They tend to take a little and wonder why they aren't losing weight.

To successfully lose weight, you have to take at least 1000 mg of carnitine per day. I recommend that you start out with 1000 and work your way up to possibly 4000. See how you are doing with the thousand for a few days then add another thousand and see how you are feeling. You will know if you need to add more. Everyone is different and your body will respond differently from someone else's. Carnitine will not hurt you. However, it may keep you awake at night; don't take it in the evening or you may be up all night.

When you are starting out, take 500 mg in the morning on an empty stomach before breakfast and the other 500 mg on an empty stomach before you eat lunch. Take no more for the rest of the day. I want you to be able to sleep at night. Remember, this nutrient does give you energy. After a few days, increase your dose to 1000 in the morning and 1000 before lunch. You can increase your dose as time goes by, but don't go over the 4000 mg dose. You don't need more than that.

HOW CARNITINE WORKS BEST

Now you aren't going to go out and buy some carnitine, take it, and do nothing else. You need to do some things to enhance it, so that it works to its best ability.

For one, carnitine works best with a diet that is low in carbohydrates, you know—sugar and starches, the junky foods you are eliminating. According to Robert Crayhon, this is because a higher intake of carbohydrates can promote an elevated level of the hormone insulin, which inhibits optimal carnitine activity. Also, eating a diet rich in omega-3 fats and increasing your intake of proteins improves carnitine's performance.

Some form of exercise is also going to help carnitine to work its best.

WHAT KIND OF CARNITINE DO I TAKE?

As you go into the health food store, you will find that there are different kinds of carnitine: L-Carnitine and Acetyl-L-Carnitine. There is D-Carnitine and DL-Carnitine, but evidently the D's are not available in the U.S., because the D-Carnitine molecule interferes with the action of the natural L-Carnitine.

But, for maximum results in weight loss, buy Tartrate Carnitine. The tartrate form works best because it is in its purest form. Carnitine Synergy is a combination of L-Carnitine-L-Tartrate and Acetyl-L-Carnitine. Carnitine Synergy is indeed the most effective for weight loss. I also recommend it especially if you are over forty. Acetyl-L-Carnitine is great for preventing Alzheimer's disease and for enhancing mental energy.

Combining these two forms will give your metabolism a boost, increase your energy level, improve weight loss, and slow the aging process!

I do want to warn you—carnitine is a little expensive. However, it is one of the most important things you can do for losing weight quickly and successfully.

CARNITINE MADE ME A BELIEVER

I was walking through the health food store, in the book department, and came across Robert Crayhon's book *The Carnitine Miracle: The Supernutrient Program that Promotes High Energy, Fat Burning, Heart Health, Brain Wellness, and Longevity*. I grabbed the book, as I am always looking for better ways to improve my health.

I was amazed by the benefits of adding this nutrient to your daily life. I stood in the store reading the book, brought it home, and the next day was back in the store to get some carnitine.

I started taking it, starting out with 1000 mg per day, 500 before breakfast and 500 before lunch. I actually felt a difference after only three days of taking it. I then increased the dose until I got to 4000 mg per day, which is what I continue to take. After the first week, I started to walk further, doubling the length of my daily walk, and shortly after that, I was doing it twice a day, walking again in the evening.

My mind became much clearer; my memory improved; I no longer had any food cravings; and the list goes on. After taking carnitine for only five weeks, I had lost twenty-two pounds. I continued to eat; I had already cut down on my carbohydrates and increased my intake of protein before I even started taking the carnitine. My diet did not change; I was already doing what the book advised me to do. Not only did I lose the weight, but I also lost cellulite! My thighs and butt smoothed out. I was actually happier about losing the cellulite than I was about the weight. (You know what I'm talking about.) Everyone noticed and was amazed by the big difference in my body. So, of course all of my friends wanted me to share with them my findings; everyone around me is now slim and trim, for they too are taking carnitine. I have people taking it that don't need to lose the weight, but need more energy or want to improve their immune system, people that simply want to improve their all-around health.

I recommend that you get Crayhon's book so that you understand carnitine and all its advantages. I am focusing on weight loss; that is what *this* book is about. His book goes into detail regarding diabetes, AIDS, and many other diseases and ailments that carnitine can either help or eliminate.

As long as carnitine is sold, I will continue to take it. I'm not looking at it as simply a way of controlling my weight, but a way of total health wellness.

chapter 9

cigarettes and weight gain

QUITTING SMOKING—IN YOUR BODY

————————Why the Weight Gain?————————

Gaining weight is one of the most distressful results for most smokers who stop smoking. I've heard many times that one of the reasons that many people won't quit smoking is because they are afraid they will gain weight.

In his book *The Amino Revolution*, Dr. Erdmann gives these reasons for the tendency to put weight on rather quickly after quitting smoking:

- For one, giving up smoking causes stress, which elicits a response from the sympathetic nervous system. One way to counter this is to eat more.

- Many people, without realizing it, eat when they are anxious—whether it is about failing their driving test or giving up smoking.
- Others use eating as a substitute for the time wasting they used to get away with by smoking. When you stop smoking, you suddenly find yourself with a lot of spare time, and it must be tempting to fill it by eating an extra snack or two.
- With your digestion improving as a result of giving up smoking, you will probably feel hungrier. You might have to eat more at mealtimes just to feel satisfied.
- Smoking creates abnormal fatty acids in your system. These fatty acids are destructive. Your body responds by manufacturing anabolic steroid output to counteract them. When you stop smoking, you stop the influx of abnormal fatty acids, but your body is still manufacturing the anabolic steroids for a while—often making it difficult for you to keep the weight off.

Erdmann says these factors tend to act on each other, sometimes making the weight gain dramatic. To prevent this from happening, many nutritionists have found amino acids to be a marvelous appetite suppressant. Aminos need to be taken in a blend rather than one amino alone, along with minerals and vitamins that complement each other. It can actually be quite dangerous to take an amino by itself. Your vitamins and minerals should be bought at a health food store, and one that is of the highest quality.

A Formula to Combat Cravings for Smoking

If you should decide to stop smoking, you can depend on amino acids to help you overcome the difficulties of the physical and mental cravings with this formula.

Amino Acids:

Phenylalanine
Tyrosine
Methionine
Glutamine
Glycine
Lysine
Carnitine

Cofactors:

Vitamin B_3
Vitamin B_6
Vitamin C
Vitamin D
Zinc

—— *PRECAUTIONS* ——

There are some precautions you need to take before taking either of these formulas. You need to take a combination because you need to work with the body as a whole, not isolating one particular area at a time. You want full health balance.

You should not take this combination if you are pregnant, taking monoamine oxidase inhibitors (MAO), or if you have difficulty metabolizing a particular amino acid. You may have trouble with metabolizing amino acids and not even realize it until you actually start taking them. If you take amino supplements and experience unpleasant physical or psy-

chological symptoms, stop taking them immediately, then take them only under the supervision of your doctor or a qualified nutritionist.

Do not give amino supplements to children or mentally retarded individuals.

It is not recommended that you give smoking up all at once; take your time. When you take this formula of amino acids along with the cofactors, they won't just help you fight the cravings, anxiety, tension, fatigue, and depression; they will also help your body recover from the biochemical damage done by smoking. Amino acid supplements will improve your physical well-being at a much higher rate and will increase your desire to give up smoking completely.

Evening primrose oil (Efamol) is something else that aids in weight control, and works great on curbing your appetite; it is also used for depression and anxiety. These two components are indeed needed for quitting smoking. Depression and anxiety will accompany your journey to becoming a nonsmoker. Last year while visiting Sweden, I recommended to a young woman that she start taking evening primrose oil to help curb her appetite while on her weight loss program. I went with her to the health food store and everyone there insisted that evening primrose oil is for PMS. Well, we take it for PMS so that we won't eat everything that is not bolted down; it also helps with the depression that accompanies PMS. So, if it does this while we are having our period, it will also work when we are not. Many doctors prescribe evening primrose oil to psychiatric patients; they also lose weight along with balancing their emotions. Take it if you are trying to kick the cigarette habit and not gain the weight.

QUITTING SMOKING—IN YOUR MIND

The hardest thing about giving up smoking is convincing yourself that you need to. Everyone knows in great detail the facts that are involved in the health issues of smoking. Smoking *kills!* We all know that; we're taught in grade school what smoking does to us. We've all seen those films on cancer related to smoking. They're enough to scare the daylights out of you. We've seen information on the news, television specials, and magazine articles. "Hazardous to your health" is on the cigarette package, yet we still buy the product. We all have someone close to us that has died from a smoking-related disease, yet we keep spending our money on cigarettes. I'm not trying to be a nag here; I'm one to talk. On occasion, I smoke cigars.

There is great power in the mind. If you believe that you are going to gain weight after you quit smoking, you will do whatever you believe. What we believe, we become. Louise Hay, in her book *You Can Heal Your Life*, teaches us that when we try to release a pattern, the whole situation seems to get worse for a while. This is a good thing. It is a sign that the situation is beginning to move. We are making affirmations; they are working; and we need to keep going.

Sometimes the problem moves in a different direction; we then begin to see and understand more. For example, you are trying to give up smoking and you are saying, "I am willing to give up the 'need' for cigarettes." As you continue to do this, you notice that your relationships are becoming more uncomfortable. This is actually a sign that the process is working.

You may ask yourself: "Am I willing to give up uncomfortable relationships? Were my cigarettes creating a smoke screen so I wouldn't see how uncomfortable these relationships are? Why am I creating these relationships?"

You notice that the cigarettes are only a symptom and not a cause. Now you are developing insight and understanding that will set you free.

You begin to say, "I am willing to release the 'need' for uncomfortable relationships." Then you notice the reason that you are so uncomfortable is that other people always seem to criticize you.

Being aware that we always create all of our experiences, you now begin to say, "I am willing to release the need to be criticized." You then think about criticism, and you realize that as a child you were always being criticized. The little kid inside you only feels "at home" when it is being criticized. Your way of hiding from this was to create a "smoke screen." Your next step would be to make the affirmation "I am willing to forgive . . ." As you continue to do your affirmations, you may find that cigarettes no longer attract you, and the people in your life no longer criticize you. Then you know that you have released your need.

Make positive affirmations and know that the thoughts you are thinking and the words you are declaring at this moment are creating your future. Making affirmations usually takes a little time to work.

If you want to quit smoking and not gain weight, or if there are any other changes you want to make in your life, go to a mirror, look into your eyes, and say out loud, "I now realize that I have created this condition, and I am now willing to release the pattern in my consciousness that is responsible for this condition." Say it several times with feeling.

Convince yourself in the mirror that this time you are ready to step out of the bondage of the past.

All you need is to be willing, you don't necessarily need to know all the how tos. The universe will figure out how to make things work. If you feel frightened because you don't know how to do the releasing, this is just resistance. Just move through it. Remember that every thought that you think and every word that you speak is being responded to by the universal intelligence of your subconscious mind. All thoughts and words are being responded to, and the power is in the moment. The thoughts you are thinking and the words you are speaking are creating your future.

chapter 10

food combining to change your metabolism

CHANGE YOUR LIFESTYLE

If you really want to lose weight, you must change your lifestyle. This really is not difficult, and once you start a new way of living, you will welcome it and only want more. When you change your eating habits, you will find that you have much more energy, are healthier, and just feel better all around. That alone will make it easy.

I also do not want this to be too painful. I want you to enjoy eating your meals. Healthy eating is nurturing yourself, loving yourself. There is no reason to starve yourself; I want you to eat and make mealtime a joyous time.

Many of you probably feel guilty when eating and think of food as a bad thing. Why? Because you may gain weight. We are going to change that. I'm going to teach you how to combine different foods for better digestion: what foods to eliminate from your diet, what foods to add, and how to have your metabolism work at an optimal level. It is possible to change your metabolism, and you do not have to diet to change it.

When I refer to diet in that way, I'm talking about starving yourself. You will be *changing* your diet, the specific foods you are consuming. So, if you read the word "diet," please don't think of this word as in taking food away. This is not a punishment! You want to be happier, live a healthier life, and feel young—full of energy. I want you to get off of the diet roller coaster, have a new lifestyle, a whole new way of eating that will change the way you think about losing weight and gaining energy.

Every food has an electromagnetic power. Every food is ready to release its power and increase your energy. Dead foods carry dead weight. There is no power to junk foods, sugars, high-starch foods like white flour and potatoes, caffeine, and alcohol. If you feel that you just have to have that piece of chocolate cake, that cherry pie—take not the whole pie, just a piece; don't punish yourself. It's okay to indulge once in a while without feeling guilty. Know that this is just a once-in-a-while thing and get back to the good stuff. Actually, once you change your lifestyle, the way you eat, the way that you think, you more than likely will not want those junk foods.

You are first going to eliminate the kinds of foods that are sugar sources. When trying to lose weight, stay completely away from sugars. Even if you don't want to lose weight and just want to be healthier, stay away from these.

Sugar Sources to Avoid

Beets	Fructose	Raw sugar
Brown Sugar	Honey	Sucrose
Carrots	Maple syrup	White sugar
Corn syrup	Molasses	

You may be wondering why avoid carrots. They are very high in natural sugar. If you think you need the vitamin A and the beta carotene, you can get the beta carotene in apricots, cantaloupe, collard greens, broccoli, and kale. You can pick up your vitamin A in cantaloupe, peaches, and apricots. Also, avoid honey where possible, but if you are going to have the ACV cocktail described elsewhere in this book, you can put a teaspoon of honey in the drink to cut the taste of the apple cider vinegar.

You don't want to give your body extra sugar; you want your body to use the fat reserves already for energy. Starch sources are the next group of junk foods for you to eliminate, because they turn into sugar once they are digested.

Starch Sources to Avoid

Bananas	Pumpkin	White rice
Corn/popcorn	Sweet potatoes	Winter squashes
Potatoes	White or semolina flour	Yams

It has been ages since I have eaten white rice. Most of you probably think that rice is good for you. Health experts say stay away from it. Eat brown rice. It tastes so much better. It has a different texture and is actually kind of nutty. As far as bananas go, once you eat them, they turn directly into sugar. If you feel you have to have a banana for the potassium, you should know that you can get it from celery, mangoes, broccoli, tomatoes, prunes, oranges, lemons, and asparagus.

Next, you should eliminate from your diet caffeinated drinks and stimulants. Consider switching to decaffeinated coffee and drinking herb teas. As we all know, beer, along with other alcohol, should be avoided, although it has been proven that some wine is beneficial to your health. By that, I don't mean go out and drink all the wine that you want, especially if you are trying to melt down.

Once you reach your goal weight, you can then work some of these foods back into your regimen. Take one day at a time and listen to your body. Your body will let you know what it needs. Hold it right there! I don't mean chocolate. (You know what I mean—"I need a chocolate fix.") If you have it, you will be up for a few minutes and then your energy level will drop very quickly.

What you should do throughout this weight loss process, and forever, is drink a lot of water—at least eight glasses a day of distilled water. However, it is recommended that you do not drink with your meals. When you are eating, your saliva mixes with your food and helps with digestion. Let your own saliva create better digestion, making sure that you are absorbing the nutrients properly.

You are also going to remove fruits from your meals. When you eat fruit, eat it as a meal in itself. Eat it a couple of hours after you have had a meal. When you eat fruit with other food, the fruit sits in your stomach and rots when combined with other food, and you lose the nutrients from both the fruit and the other foods. This can leave you feeling pretty lousy, with an upset stomach, gas, bloating, and an acidic stomach.

If you are low in energy, do not have milk with meat. Even the Bible says so. Milk neutralizes the stomach acid that meat needs to be digested. So, meat with milk will sit in your stomach and decay. Besides that, meat and milk neutralize the electromagnetic pattern, creating a complete void.

Fat-free food is not going to guarantee that you will lose weight. Fat-free cookies for example are still junk food—empty of any nutritional value and just a filler. They leave your body nutritionally unsatisfied and hungry for a decent meal. These fat-free foods still contain sugar; we get fat because we eat too much sugar. Sugar, in my opinion, is the body's worst enemy.

FOOD COMBINING

For a healthy digestion, we need to separate protein meals from carbohydrate meals. According to Hanna Kroeger, author of many health-related books, grains and proteins should definitely be separated. Do not eat these foods together.

Vegetables above the ground, combined with grains, release an enormous amount of energy and the body is able to absorb every bit of it. Also, vegetables above the ground, combined with protein, become a super charger.

Vegetables below the ground, combined with protein (like a meal of meat and potatoes), release only a fair amount of energy.

Grains with fruit juice build mucus in the stomach and nullify the energy patterns of these two foods.

Grains and protein, taken at the same time, nullify the electromagnetic power completely.

Kroeger also says that God placed fruit on the trees and vegetables on the ground so we would not mix them at the same meal. When we eat them together, we have no energy. As I said, the fruit rots in your stomach and destroys any nutritional value that you could have been receiving from these foods.

I know that it sounds awful to give up sugar and starches, and it may even be difficult, but know that it is only temporary. Well, I would like to see you stay away from sugar for the rest of your life! Once you get down to the weight you are wishing for, then you can have sugar and starches in moderation. Occasionally, splurge, but you will be feeling so good without it that you won't even want to bring it back into your diet.

Every once in a while I want to have chocolate. For some reason I feel that I need it or deserve it. One day, I wanted a break and decided I would walk over to the drugstore and get myself some M&Ms. Of course I bought one of those big bags. I don't normally eat sugar, not to mention candy, period. I filled my hand with those tiny, mouth-melting bits of chocolate, and popped them into my mouth, filling it as though they were going to be taken away from me. Then I felt kind of sick to my stomach. Maybe I should have just eaten a few. I thought I would eat them up, get them out of the way, so there would be no more to eat and I wouldn't be tempted to eat them because they would all be gone.

I'm sure many of you know exactly what I'm talking about. You go out and buy those Oreo cookies and sit down to eat them all at once to get them gone so that there will be no more for you to eat, so you don't get fat.

Well, back to my M&Ms: one handful, I now feel sick, don't need anymore; I don't even want any more and I wonder why I felt that I had to have them. By not having them was I depriving myself of something I thought I wanted, that I really didn't want? Oh well, I got it out of my system and threw the rest of them into the trash. Now I could have saved them and given them to the next person who visited me, but then I would be telling them that it's okay to eat that junk. Everyone knows I stay clear of those kinds of foods. Yeah, right! M&Ms are food! Well, I'm only human and will not feel guilty for eating them. I'm being punished enough; I have a stomachache. But they did taste kind of good!

What I should have done was had maybe ten pieces of candy and my desire for those little morsels would have been satisfied. And that is all right; do things in moderation. If I had done that, I would have been satisfied, but no, I had to be a glutton. And that too shall pass. That's a phrase I like to use when things do not seem well. I simply say, "And this too shall pass!"

There's another thing I do when there is something I really don't want to put into my body, but there's a part of me saying, "I have to have it!" I tell myself that it tastes bad to me and that I really do not want it. Try it. You are telling your unconscious mind that you don't want it or need it. Your unconscious mind will listen and trigger whatever it is that you are making your belief system, and let your conscious mind know what it is that you need to do. This may not make sense to you. If you tell yourself what it is that you want your belief system to be, it does get triggered, and it will become your belief system.

You become and are whatever it is that you believe that you are. If you believe you are the unluckiest person there is, as long as you believe that, you will be unlucky. If you believe that you are and there is no way out, that's more than likely exactly what will come into being. So . . . not only are you changing your weight, but you are also changing your lifestyle and how you view yourself, how you feel about you.

We will get into this more in another chapter. However, before I get out of this I want to give you an example of what I'm saying and how you can change your belief system. This has nothing to do with food combining, but we are going there anyway. When I was in Sedona, Arizona, a few years back, I was working on my book, *Mind Travelers*. I was to interview someone for the book and found he had an intuitive message for me: stop driving through the fast-food place drinking that junk. Well, this was the first time this man had ever met me; he did not know about my diet cola addiction. I'm serious, this was a big addiction.

I would drive through a fast-food place about seven times a day and order the biggest size they had. This stuff is really bad for you, and here I was filling myself with it daily, not to mention spending a fortune on it. I was also doing it secretly; I didn't want anyone to know that this really was a problem for me. I never bought it to have at home, but I would be driving along and it would be as if my car had a mind of its own, like its autopilot would come on. I would drive the car into a fast-food place if I didn't already have a soda. Often I would have a cup about a quarter full and would have to get one for when it was empty. I became a regular at a couple of places that started giving them to me free, or they would charge me in the morning for the first one and the rest of them for the day were on the house.

Well, back to this interview. He told me that I was killing myself by drinking this junk, and that I needed to stop. I didn't discuss it with him, neither admitting it nor denying it. I left his home, went around the corner, saw a fast-food restaurant, and drove through. I sat there in line telling myself that I did not want this; I was wasting money and my body. I'm a firm believer in what I teach, so I said to myself, "I do not want this and it will taste bad to me." I drove up, ordered my large diet cola, took one taste, and it tasted bad to me. I pulled over, poured it out, and didn't have the urge for one for about a year. Even then when I had one, there was no urge for it and after drinking it, I didn't want another soda. I drink it occasionally today, but I would prefer water or tea, something that is going to make me feel good. My point—you can conquer any dragon! Diet cola, and the thought that I had to have it, was my dragon.

Let's get back to food combining! In all the research I have been doing for years, I have found a great deal of information about food combinations, with most experts agreeing on the same combinations. There are small different twists with some. However, the information I am about to give contains the most commonly used and taught food combinations.

In Suzanne Somers's book, *Eat Great, Lose Weight,* she teaches about food combining and offers wonderful recipes and meals to help you eat in a healthy way and lose weight. She teaches you to eat. All experts want you to eat. She calls her system "Somersizing."

If you starve yourself of food, you starve yourself of nutrients, slow down your metabolism, and you won't lose weight. You also become malnourished, which thousands of Americans are. In depriving yourself of healthy foods and nutrition, you create disease. It is my intention to encourage you to be healthy, lose weight, and rid yourself of disease or possible illness that can come about because you are not taking proper care of yourself.

CARBOHYDRATES

There are two different kinds of carbohydrates: refined carbohydrates and complex carbohydrates. Refined carbs are the ones in junk foods, like white flour, sugar, the ones I want you to avoid. We will not be combining this carb with any food group. Carbohydrates are derived from plant rather than animal sources.

Complex carbs contain essential vitamins and nutrients and provide fiber necessary for the digestive process. However, you want to keep your carbohydrates low in your diet; try not to eat too many of them if you are trying to lose weight. When I speak of eating carbohydrates, I'm speaking about complex carbs, never the refined ones. You can combine carbs with one another or combine them with vegetables.

Beans and nonfat dairy products are actually proteins, but because they are high in carbohydrates and the way your body reacts to them, we are putting them in with the carbs.

Beans and Grains (Combine with Vegetables)

There are many kinds of beans; try ones that maybe you have never eaten. Experiment with them. Of the grains, spelt is especially great if you have a problem with your thyroid working properly or have any yeast conditions *(Candida albicans)*.

Beans		
Adzuki	Garbanzo	Peas, green
Anasazi	Kidney	Pinto
Black	Lentils	Red
Black-eyed peas	Lima	Split peas
Cannellini	Mung	
Fava	Navy	

Grains		
Amaranth barley	Crackers	Rice (brown)
Bagels	Kamut	Rye
Breads (no white bread)	Millet	Spelt
Buckwheat	Mustards (brown, Dijon, whole-grain, and yellow)	Wheat
Bulgar	Oats	Wheat germ
Cereals (hot and cold)	Pasta	Wild rice

Nonfat Dairy Products

Cheeses	Cream cheese	Sour cream
Cottage cheese	Milk	Yogurt

VEGETABLES AND HERBS (Combine with Proteins/Fats Alone or Carbohydrates Alone)

Vegetables can be eaten alone, with proteins/fats, or with carbohydrates.

First, a note about avocados: Some believe we should eliminate them from our diet. I disagree completely! The avocado requires no spraying with poisonous chemicals because the tree is strong and insects leave it alone. It has unsaturated fats that the body can handle easily and has more potassium than banana! Make some guacamole with it by mushing it up, add slices of tomatoes, celery, radishes, cucumber, red and green bell peppers, a little lemon juice . . . you have a wonderfully delicious, high-vibrational lunch.

Tomatoes are included here, although they are a fruit. They work with your body more like a vegetable. Now, for the rest of the vegetable and herbs list.

Alfalpha sprouts	Dandelion greens	Radishes
Artichokes	Dill	Rhubard Sag

Arugula	Eggplant	Rosemary
Asparagus	Endive	Sage
Avocados	Escarole	Salsify
Bamboo shoots	Fennel	Sauerkraut
Basil	Garlic	Shallots
Bean sprouts	Ginger	Snow Peas
Beet greens	Green beans	Spinach
Bok choy	Horseradish	Sugar snap peas
Broccoli	Kale	Swiss chard
Brussel sprouts	Kohlrabi	Tarragon
Cabbage	Leeks	Thyme
Cauliflower	Lettuce	Tomatillo
Celery	Mushrooms	Tomato
Chervil	Mustard greens	Tomato greens
Chicory	Okra	Turnip
Chives	Onions	Turnip greens
Cilantro	Parsley	Watercress
Clover sprouts	Parsnips	Wax bens
Collard greens	Peppers	Yard-long beans
Crookneck squash	Pickles (not sweet)	Zucchini
Cucumber	Purslane	
Daikon	Radicchio	

Many proteins contain fat; therefore, fats are included in this group.

Cheeses

American	Feta	Mozzarella
Asiago	Fontina	Parmesan
Babybel	Goat	Pecorino
Bel Paese	Gruyère	Provolone
Blue	Havarti	Queso blanco
Brie	Hoop	Ricotta
Camembert	Jarlsberg	Romano
Cheddar	Limburger	Roquefort
Colby	Mascarpone	Swiss
Farmer	Monterey Jack	

Other Dairy Products

Butter	Eggs	Mayonnaise
Cream	Margarine	Sour cream

PROTEINS/FATS (Combine with Vegetables)

Eliminate margarine from your diet. When you eat margarine, once it is in your system, the way it looks in the tub or stick is how it is going to look in your body, your blood. It simply goes back to its original form. Butter may be higher in fat, but in the long run is much better for you. I haven't eaten margarine in years and plan to keep it that way!

Fish

Anchovies	Halibut	Sea Bass
Bass	HerrinMackerelg	Shark
Bluefish	Mahimahi	Smelt
Bonito	Monkfish	Snapper
Burbot	Ocean perch	Sole
Carp	Organce roughy	Sturgeon
Catfish	Pollock	Swordfish
Cod	Pompano	Trout
Eel	Red Snapper	Tuna
Flat fish	Sablefish	Turbot
Flounder	Salmon	Whitefish
Gefilte fish	Sardines	Wolf fish

Grouper		Yellowtail
Haddock		

Meat

Bacon	Ham	Pork
Beef	Lamb	Rabbit
Canadian bacon	Pastrami	Veal
Frog legs	Pepperoni	Venison

I have left lunchmeats (cold cuts), hot dogs, and sausage off this list. You may want to consider not eating ham and meats like that. I've put in all of the above because the public eats these foods, not that I am recommending that you eat them. Do your homework then decide what meats you want to eat. I eat some red meat, poultry, and fish. I stay away from bacon, ham, cold cuts, etc.

Oils

Chili oil	Peanut oil	Sesame oil
Corn oil	Safflower oil	Vegetable oil
Olive oil		

I recommend you use olive oil on a daily basis. I take a tablespoon of olive oil every day, often as much as three times a day. It aids in cleansing your system and keeping your colon clean.

Poultry

Capon	Goose	Quail
Chicken	Guinea hen	Squab
Cornish hen	Pheasant	Turkey
Duck		

Seafood

Abalone	Crayfish	Octopus
Caviar	Lobster	Scallops
Clams	Mussels	Shrimp
Crab		Squid

FRUITS (Eat Alone, No Combinations)

Apple	Lemon	Pear
Apricot	Lime	Persimmon
Asian pear	Loquat	Pineapple

Berries	Mandarin oranges	Plum
Cherries	Mango	Pomegranate
Crabapple	Melon	Pomelo
Fig	Nectarine	Prickly pear
Grapefruit	Orange	Quince
Grapes	Papaya	Star fruit
Guava	Passion fruit	Tangelo
Kiwi	Peach	Tangerine
Kumquat		

Remember, you are going to eat fruits alone! I hate to repeat myself, but it is important to eat them alone. Wait at least an hour before or after a meal to eat your fruit.

It's best to try not to eat the same foods often. Rotate your different foods. I know that often we have our favorites and tend to eat certain foods frequently, sometimes several days in a row. If you switch them around, you get a better balance of nutrition and you won't be apt to develop an allergy to foods. When you eat a food too often, it is easy to develop an allergy to that food.

So . . .here is what you are going to do:

Cut out the junk foods
Eliminate from your diet white sugar, white flour, packaged and processed foods, and margarine
Eat fruits alone and on an empty stomach
Eat proteins and fats with veggies
Eat carbohydrates with veggies and no fat
Keep proteins and fats separate from carbohydrates

It is very important not to miss any meals. Eat slowly; enjoy your meal; chew, chew, chew. If you take your time, you will be less apt to overeat and will digest your food much better. Don't drink anything with your meal unless you are going to have a small glass of wine on occasion. Between meals, drink a lot of water, at least eight to ten glasses. Often when you feel hungry, what your body is really telling you to do is to feed it fluids; you may just be thirsty.

Again, do not miss any meals. To lose weight you need to speed up your metabolism. If you in fact starve yourself or crash diet, you will lose weight, but when you start eating, you will gain it back again. It's also very dangerous to stop eating, especially if you have any health problems.

Once you lose the desired weight, you might want to start eating differently. This means eating when your body tells you it is hungry. You don't have to eat at noon just because it is expected for that time of the day. Don't eat out of boredom or loneliness.

Don't forget to get some exercise while you are developing a new lifestyle. A little exercise will help you speed up your metabolism.

Be easy on yourself!

chapter 11

love and sex

Love is always the answer to healing of any sort.

Being in love feels so wonderful, it truly makes you feel good; it makes life much easier and helps eliminate stress. And, of course, we all know that sex is a great stress reducer, good exercise, and creates other benefits for your body, mind, and spirit.

But you need most of all to love yourself, to love yourself in a healthy way. Love is a miracle cure, and loving ourselves works miracles in our lives.

I'm not talking about vanity or arrogance, being stuck-up; that is not love. That is only fear. I am talking about having a great respect for ourselves and a gratitude for the miracle of our bodies and our minds.

If we deny our good in any way, it is an act of not loving ourselves. Lack of self-worth is another expression of not loving ourselves.

How many times have you run into someone that you haven't seen in a while to find that they have lost weight? I'm talking about a lot of weight. Of course you have to mention that they look terrific, full of life, full of passion; there is a special glow about them. You ask them how they did it. They then answer that they are in love. They have met that special someone and have fallen in love; they have never been happier and it shows.

Being in love brought incredible happiness to me. Yes, all the delicious sex, lovemaking, whatever you are going to call it, does indeed promote weight loss. Not just the act itself, although it is great exercise. I remember hearing years ago that having sex was equivalent to a five-mile run. I don't know if that is actually true but I'll buy it.

However, the intimacy, the touching, the loving, is all so very important in being healthy. Even if you are not in a sexual relationship, you need to be touched and to be touching others. I'm talking about hugging those that you care about, telling people that you love—your parents, your children, your partner—that you love them. You have to be loving and giving to be able to receive love and to love yourself.

Loving yourself is the most important key to being healthy. If you love yourself, you will only be kind to yourself, not punish yourself. You will take care of yourself the best way you can. You will nurture yourself and want only to treat yourself gently, nurture yourself, and give yourself the best treatment that you can receive in body, mind, and spirit.

When you love, you feel alive, happy, and warm inside. Even if the other person is not receiving your love, if you continue loving, you reap love's benefits. Remember when you were very young and in love? You had a "boyfriend" or a "girlfriend," only the other person didn't know that they were your boyfriend or girlfriend. I remember when I was young and someone would ask, "Do you have a boyfriend?" Of course I would reply, "Yes, his name is Bob." The only problem was that while I was in love with Bob, and I called him my boyfriend, he didn't know anything about it. So . . . he wasn't receiving my love. But it felt delicious to be in love. It had nothing to do with him loving me back; it just felt good to be loving. As adults, if you can recapture that feeling and not be afraid to love, you will be happier and healthier.

The problem is that when people do something you don't like, it becomes difficult for you to continue loving them, and so you stop loving them. Then you feel hurt. The deepest hurt in your life is when you withdraw your love from others.

Love connects you to the power within you. That's why it feels so good to be in love. When you stop loving others, you weaken your connection to your inner power and your ability to love yourself. You always win by loving, because that experience of loving is nourishing you and empowering you. If you are not going to allow yourself to love because maybe someone has hurt you, you are going to lack that nourishment; we often replace that emotion with nourishing ourselves with food.

Remember, this doesn't just pertain to being in romantic love, but in loving all others. Maybe your mother or your father hurt you and you were unable to give love after that because you related loving with pain. So, now you withhold from others.

Check out your emotional self. If you are in need of some counsel, I highly recommend that you seek some. Are you having problems with repeating patterns? Are you using food in place of receiving love or loving yourself, giving love? Get emotional help so that you can be happy, healthy, and loving.

I believe you should have passion for everything you do—passion in loving, in making love, in your work, and in life itself. Passion will keep you young, alive, and, therefore, will keep you fit because you will want to take care of yourself.

For some reason, some people sit down and begin to deteriorate, age. I don't believe you have to stop living. As long as you have a healthy mind, you can have a healthy body. Then there is always the topic of sex and the aging. For some odd reason, many think that when you get older, your sex drive shuts down. I believe that a sexually active life and passion will keep you young. Keep passion in loving, passion for your work, passion for your interests, such as hobbies—simply passion for life. If you can keep a young mind, stay in some way childlike, you will stay young and healthy.

I spoke with my father not too long ago about his sex life. My father is 87 years old. My mother passed away a few years ago and he now has a girlfriend. Last year I was in California visiting when he and his girlfriend kept bringing up at different times that they needed to clean the refrigerator. I was thinking that he must have the cleanest refrigerator in town. I finally figured out that that was their signal to go make love. I asked my dad if he was still sexually active. He said of course he was, that God had given him the ability and that he would use it "as often as I can." You go, Daddy.

My father plays golf, goes rattlesnake hunting, and loves life. I think he also thinks he is still forty years old. He refuses to give up and grow old. His attitude about life, sex, loving, romance, and passion is refreshing and he is proof that your frame of mind has everything to do with being healthy and being young. Dr. Papon, asked to name the most important ingredient for permanent weight loss, said that the best way to lose weight and to keep it off is to fall in love!

When you have healthy thoughts and attitudes toward sex and loving, such is the stuff of heaven.

chapter 12

heal your life through visualization

Thought is energy and energy creates energy. What we believe about ourselves and about life becomes true for us. When we create peace, harmony, and balance in our minds, we will find it in our lives.

No matter what your problems are, your experiences are just outer effects of inner thoughts. "I'm fat. I'm ugly. I'm a bad person." These thoughts produce a feeling, and you buy into that feeling. However, if you don't have that thought, you won't have that feeling. Thoughts can be changed; change the thought and the feeling must go.

It doesn't matter how long we have had a negative pattern. The point of the power is in the present moment. We can begin to be free in this moment! Often we think the same thought for so long that it does not seem as though we are choosing it. It becomes a habit. We made the original choice; we can refuse certain thoughts now. How many times have you refused a positive thought? It is just as easy to refuse a negative thought. How many times has someone given you a compliment and you cringed? I've done it, so I know that you have or most of you have. Start accepting compliments. Know that you are a good person; you do deserve all the deliciousness of life. Start believing in yourself. You are beautiful.

Besides being an author and health researcher, I am also a photographer. Years ago a woman called me to take her portrait. She needed a picture of herself, thin. She weighed 169 pounds. She had lost weight, her highest point having been about 425 pounds. She had very nearly died three times because she was so fat, so big. Once her heart had failed her. Another time it was because her own fecal matter, which had built up in her over a period of three weeks, had actually poisoned her.

Evidently she wasn't ready to go, because she came back. Well—when you die three times and you come back each time, I would say it's time to say *no* more. She really didn't care about her life until this last event. It made her think that God was giving her another chance and she had better do something about it. For her to just stop eating, to diet, was quite a challenge. She had not left her home in three years, just stayed in the house and ate.

She knew she had to call on some higher help, call on her spirit to help her, as we are not one entity—we are body, mind, and spirit. By calling on our spirit, we are calling on our power within, the God within. She went from 425 pounds to 169 by meditating, by visualizing herself being strong, visualizing herself thin and healthy. She made affirmations about losing weight, saying that she was not hungry, that she was losing weight and it was easy, and that she was happy and healthy. This worked for her so well that she ended up opening several obesity clinics.

We have to reprogram our minds as she did, speak to our higher selves, tell our higher selves what we believe, our new thought patterns. Yes, you look in the mirror every day and say it out loud. Tell the universe what it is that you are choosing for yourself—a new belief system.

I am beautiful.
I am forever young.
I am filled with love and affection.
I love myself.
I am totally healthy.
I do not want sugar.
I have a lot of energy.
Illness cannot attach itself to me.
I am now in a healthy relationship.
I am prosperous.
I forgive _____ (Name the person; say it out loud; forgive everyone who has hurt you. This is a very powerful exercise!)

You will now learn to think in positive affirmations.

YOUR MIND

You probably believe that your mind controls you. The truth is *you* control your mind. You choose what comes in and what goes out. Your body responds to your thoughts and your words. You can stop thinking those old thoughts, the unworthy thoughts. "I am not smart enough. I am not pretty enough. I am fat. I am ugly. I'm simply not enough."

When your mind says that, it is hard to change your ways, to change your way of thinking, take mental control. Say to your mind, "I now choose to believe it is becoming easier for me to make changes."

Take a look at your body. Is it healthy? Are you overweight? Notice how much you hold on. The illness and the weight is negativity. If you are holding it with your body, you are holding it with your mind.

Negativity only creates more of what you do not want. Whatever you are focused on is what you will create. What you have the most resistance to is what you will create.

Self-approval and self-acceptance are the keys to positive changes. This means *no* criticism whatsoever. Are you objecting to this? You *are* going to love yourself.

Louise Hay teaches us that for every problem there is a probable cause and gives you a new thought pattern to counteract the old one and change your life. She says that if you are fat—overweight—the probable cause is oversensitivity. This often represents fear and shows a need for protection. Fear may be a cover for hidden anger and resistance to forgiveness.

Your new thought pattern is

I am protected by divine love.
I am always safe and secure.
I am willing to grow up and take responsibility for my life.
I forgive others, and I now create my own life the way I want it.
I am safe.

When you are driving along in your car or looking in the mirror, say to yourself, or out loud, that you are very proud of yourself for your accomplishments and that you are a good person. Remember that you deserve the best and tell yourself that you are healthy and beautiful. Say "I am slender and I am happy with who I am." If you feel resistance to these thoughts, say them again; say them three times. You will believe these new thoughts and then your life will change. Life is filled with deliciousness and you deserve to taste every bit of it.

MEDITATION

Do you know how to meditate? A meditation exercise will help you create what it is that you are now choosing. You want a healthy body. You want to rid yourself of unwanted weight. You want to let go of disease. You simply want to release negative energy. Negative energy is thought, we are going to release it all.

GETTING STARTED

Sit in a chair with both feet flat on the floor. You want it to be very quiet or put on some soft meditational music. Start with your toes, relaxing them, sending this relaxation slowly throughout your entire body, relaxing and letting go of all negativity, letting go of all pain, anger, hurt feelings. Let go of it all.

Let your mind go and imagine all this energy being released from the palms of your hands, the bottoms of your feet, and from the top of your head. You can feel this energy pouring from your body, releasing and letting go.

When you feel that you have let go of it all, when you feel clear, imagine a white light. Breathe this light into your body. It is pure light, pure positive energy. Fill your entire being with this energy, knowing that it is all healing. Sit and bask in this light, in this energy.

Now open your eyes and know that you have begun to live your life in a way you may have never experienced before.

This exercise should be done daily. By meditating and letting go of negativity, we can now fill ourselves with nothing but good. We can be happy, healthy, and prosperous.

If meditating is difficult for you, or if you have difficulty in focusing and would like a guided meditation, try my audiocassette tapes, *The Practical Art of Magick: Creating Your Own Reality.* I have a guided meditation where I guide you through the process of letting go and creating new energy. My address is at the back of the book. You can also purchase meditation tapes at your local music store or New Age bookstore.

chapter 13

gentle exercise

Exercise—you have to do it if you want to be healthy, if you want to lose weight. I exercise daily, but I'm far from being an exercise freak. I don't believe in the "no pain, no gain" theory. I also do not believe you have to go to a gym and beat yourself up to get a good workout. I'm not saying not to go to a gym. For many people, if they were not going to a gym, they simply would not get any exercise whatsoever. For those of you who want to exercise privately, I'm with you. Your body, mind, and spirit need you to stay in shape physically. To lose any weight, you have to get your body moving. One of the main reasons people get old is that they don't get up and move. They wait, instead of dealing with weight! Get off your butt and move. If you want to get your metabolism up, you have to move your body. If you want your thyroid to work, you have to get some exercise. If you want your metabolism to be up, you have to exercise. If you don't feel you have time in your hectic schedule to exercise, make time. By exercising, you will actually be more energized so that you can accomplish more. You will feel invigorated and want to take even better care of yourself, put better foods into your mouth. You will have more stamina for your busy schedule.

You can do many things for exercise. If you have health problems that prevent you from moving your body much, you may want to look at the section about yoga. There are yoga exercises that many people in wheelchairs can do. Yoga is wonderful for you in the body, mind, and spirit connection. It is a very gentle way to exercise.

You can do very simple things throughout the day to help create more exercise. For one, when you go to work, park your car farther away from your job. If you have to park in a large parking lot, instead of trying to park as close to work as you can, park so that you will have to walk a little farther. Instead of using the elevator, climb the stairs. At lunchtime, take a quick walk around the block. If you need incentive, think about the new figure you will have by doing some simple exercise.

Are you one of those people who have a hard time sticking to it? Get a neighbor to walk with you so that you have support, or do as I did and get a dog that depends on you for a walk. If you are at work, get someone you work with to take that stroll with you on your lunch break. Keep in mind that, for it to do any good, you have to walk like you mean it. Walk fast, swing those arms!

Take up a sport you think you may enjoy. I play golf on occasion. There is a lot of walking involved, and you swing your body. Sometimes I'll have no one to play with, or don't have the time to play nine or eighteen holes, so I will go and get a couple of baskets of balls and just go to the range and hit balls. That is great fun. Try your hand at bowling or swimming. Find something you like to do and stick with it.

Check out my section on how to belly dance. It is great exercise, makes you feel feminine and sexy, and you will work up a sweat. Do it; it's great fun and it doesn't feel like you are doing exercise.

If you are doing the speed walking or jogging and the weather does not permit, stand in front of a window and run in place.

Another thing you may want to consider is treating yourself. If you can afford it, go to a massage therapist and get yourself a full body massage. If you can do this once a week, it will really help you lose weight. Your circulation will improve and with better circulation, your blood flow will break up fat tissue. If you can't afford it regularly, do it on an occasional basis and buy yourself a book on massage. You and your mate can also massage each other. This can be great fun—you're getting your massage and getting close to your partner. If you are alone, you can massage yourself.

Get on the floor before you go to bed and try some simple stretching. Breathe deeply through your nose, not your mouth. Breathe deeply; get oxygen into your body, into your cells. This is not difficult, but most people do not breathe properly.

Last but not least, here is some real motivation. Take off your clothes, get your meal, and stand in front of a mirror and eat. I can't think of better motivation. Try it; you'll see what I mean!

YOGA

No matter what your physical condition, your age, your disabilities, or your abilities, yoga uses what you have, and makes you better.

Yoga is an ancient art that began in India before the birth of Christ. Although there are many branches of yoga, "hatha yoga" is the branch that has swept across America, offering a totally different concept of physical fitness.

The word "yoga" means union; "ha," means sun; and "tha" means moon. "Hatha Yoga" means a balanced union—a system for creating the balanced well-being of the total person. Yoga joins body, mind, and spirit into a balanced whole.

Keep in mind that yoga is not a religion and has nothing to do with religion, nor does it have anything to do with yogurt. It also has nothing to do with magic. It is a very practical system for improving life. Yoga will change you, physically and mentally.

———————— Rules to Remember ————————

- Always breathe through the nose, don't be afraid to breathe deeply. The mouth is for eating and talking.
- Don't get discouraged. Don't try to do something that you cannot do. Be easy on yourself. With practice, you will be able to do these exercises more easily.
- Don't strain yourself or practice until exhaustion.
- Practice with an empty stomach.

For most of you, this may be very new to you or some of you may have health problems that make exercising something that may be difficult for you to do. There is much more to yoga than I have included in this book. I have given you exercises that even those in a wheelchair can do. If you have any limits, you may want to get someone to help you. For example, for the shoulder stand, get someone to hold your legs up for you or get up against a wall to hold your legs up.

If you feel you would like to learn more about this gentle, healing approach to exercise and better health, I suggest you go and buy yourself a book on yoga or maybe a video. There are many on the market. What I am giving you is very basic.

Always do some breathing exercises to start out with and do all of the standing exercises first.

Breathe

When you first start this, you may want to lie on your back and place a book or your hand on your abdomen. After you have mastered this, you can do this exercise sitting up, then standing. Do what is most comfortable for you.

Be sure that you are breathing in fresh and clean air. This exercise will energize you throughout your day. Relax as you focus on how you are breathing. It helps to close your eyes.

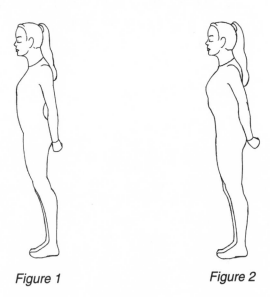

Figure 1　　　　　　　　*Figure 2*

The Pose

Figure 1. Inhale as you stretch the abdomen outward. Exaggerate this movement at first, breathing through the nostrils in an even, steady manner.

Figure 2. Follow each inhalation with an exhalation, pressing in and back with the abdominal muscles.

Your shoulders and chest should not be moving as you are breathing. Concentrate on directing energy to the solar plexus, recharging and revitalizing the body.

"Ha" Squat

This is an excellent exercise with which to begin your yoga practice. It stretches and opens the hip joints and also relieves tension in the lower back.

Feel the stretch along the backs of the legs. It strengthens and stretches the Achilles tendons, and strengthens the muscles in the front of the legs.

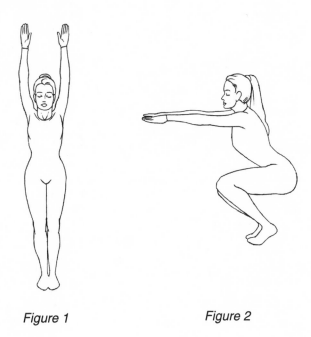

Figure 1   *Figure 2*

The Pose

Figure 1. Stand with feet placed under the hips, arms high. Inhale as you stretch your arms up, stuff the body with fresh air.

Figure 2. As you squat, blow out the stale air through your mouth.

Inhale as you stand; rest and repeat. If you cannot keep your balance, hold a chair or doorknob. You can do this with a partner, facing you and holding hands.

Chest Expander

This is great for posture alignment, and unkinking the chest, shoulders, spine, and legs. It is great if you have any back or shoulder problems.

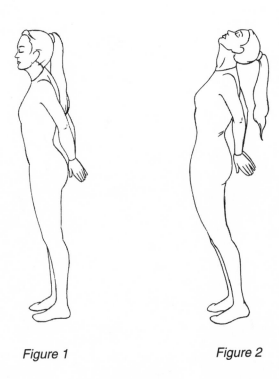

Figure 1   Figure 2

The Pose

Figure 1. Stand straight and relaxed. Feet should be a few inches apart. Bring palms together behind you and interlace fingers, keeping your arms as straight as you can.

Figure 2. Slowly bend your head back and, if it feels right, arch your back gently. Push downward with your hands.

You should feel more balanced, more straight, and you may feel tension being released from the arms and shoulders.

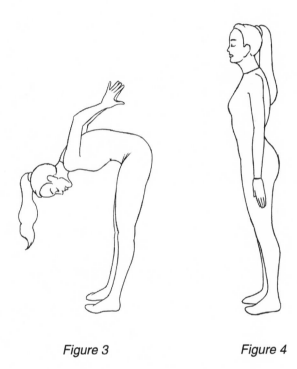

Figure 3   *Figure 4*

Figure 3. Slowly return to an erect position, begin exhaling, and bend forward from the hips. Lift your arms as far up as you can.

Figure 4. Straighten to an upright position with the next inhale breath. Release the hands; relax the neck and shoulders.

Forward Bend

This pose is vital for spinal flexibility. It promotes suppleness of the spine, tones the abdominal organs, and decreases abdominal fat and bloating.

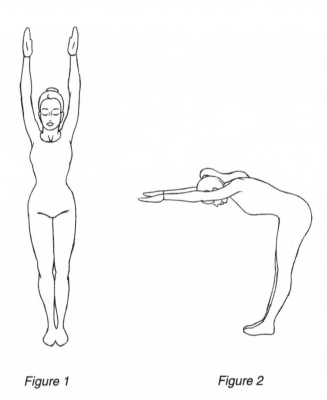

Figure 1   Figure 2

The Pose

Figure 1. Stand straight. Raise the arms with a deep inhale.

Figure 2. Stretch well, as the raised arms reach forward and then down, leading the body into its descent. Do not round your back; remain slightly concave. For those with disc problems, only go halfway.

The backs of the legs can get an intense stretch.

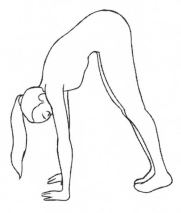

Figure 3

Figure 3. Let your body fall forward, relaxing the arms, shoulders, and back and reaching for the floor. If your fingers touch the floor, don't push yourself if you cannot go any farther. Remain in the stretch position for several seconds. If you pull the abdomen in toward the spine, you will increase your stretch.

Twisting Triangle Pose

This will give you hip and torso flexibility, elongation of the spine, and stronger, more flexible feet, ankles, knees, and legs.

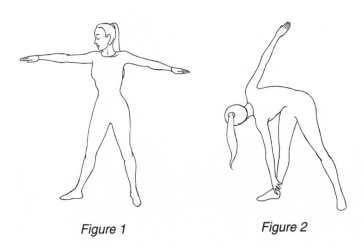

Figure 1   *Figure 2*

The Pose

Figure 1. Stand with feet three feet apart, feet placement at 30- and 90-degree angles, and arms out at shoulder height. Inhale and rotate the upper body around in a good twist.

Figure 2. Stretch out and elongate the spine; bend forward and rest the opposite hand on the extended leg. The free arm is extended upward, with the face turned toward it so that you can see your thumb. Breathe as you hold the pose.

Revolve out of the pose slowly. Rest. Then do the other side.

The Lift

This pose strengthens the wrists, ankles, legs, buttocks, and the back.

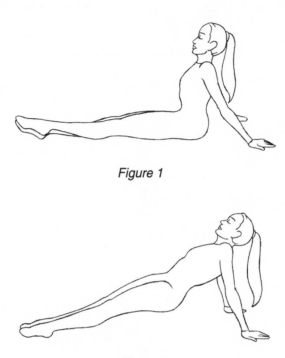

Figure 1

Figure 2

The Pose

Figure 1. Sit with legs extended and arms placed behind you, with fingers pointed outward.

Figure 2. With an inhale breath, press the feet flat and lift the hips to an incline plane. Let the head hang back, and squeeze and press the buttocks high. Hold for a breath or two. Then simply sit down with an exhalation.

Spinal Twist

A pleasant stretch and massage are felt in the hips, waist, abdomen, and internal organs. Circulation is increased around the kidneys and the intestines. It is also an aid in reducing abdominal fat and slimming the waistline.

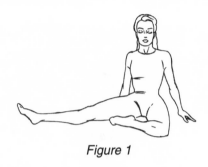

Figure 1

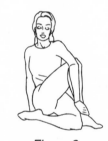

Figure 2

The Pose

Figure 1. Sit erect, legs extended and your weight directly over your sitting bones. Fold the left leg.

Figure 2. Cross your right foot over the outside of your left thigh. Inhale and exhale, rotate the trunk 90 degrees to the right, keeping the shoulders level. Bring the left arm alongside the outer side of the upraised knee. Stretch the right arm around the back, placing the palm of your hand on the floor behind your seat.

Hold, breathing shallowly. Release and repeat on the other side.

Cobra

Tones the entire back, expands the rib cage, stretches the front of the chest and abdomen, firms the throat, and bathes the pelvis and lower back with a fresh supply of blood. This gives your spine a wonderful supply of energy and promotes better mobility and circulation.

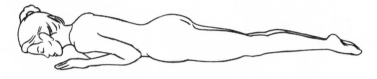

Figure 1

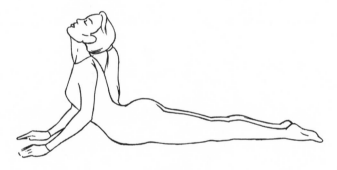

Figure 2

The Pose

Figure 1. Lie face down. Stretch the body long as you firm the buttocks and bring the feet together.

Figure 2. Curl the upper body as you raise your head, shoulders, and chest with an inhale breath. Let the spine lift you as much as it can without using the arms. Stop at a maximum point of stretch. Breathe. Slowly uncurl; descend with grace and control.

Shoulder Stand

This pose is not recommended to be practiced by persons with glaucoma or uncontrolled high blood pressure. Do not turn your head from side to side while in the posture.

This posture benefits all parts of the body. It strengthens arms, chest, and shoulders; slims legs and hips; and strengthens the back and abdominal muscles. It rejuvenates the thyroid and parathyroid glands, which regulate body weight and metabolism by natural mechanisms. There are many other benefits to this exercise, including benefit to those with varicose veins.

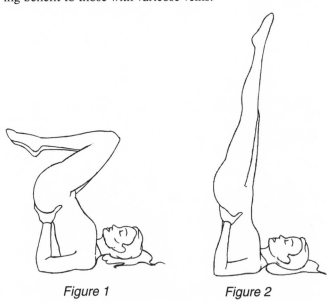

Figure 1   Figure 2

The Pose

Figure 1. Lie on your back; bend the knees; roll the hips up.

Figure 2. Place the hands lower on the trunk as you raise your legs upward. Stretch your legs high and try to straighten the back. Hold 20 to 30 seconds.

Plough

This exercise is very similar to the shoulder stand in that it helps in the same way.

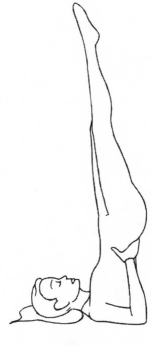

Figure 1

The Pose

Figure 1. Lie flat on your back, bringing legs up. Like the shoulder stand, place your arms on the floor, holding your lower back.

It is also therapeutic for back problems, constipation, tightness of the neck and hamstrings, glandular imbalances, abdominal fat, and "hangover" headaches.

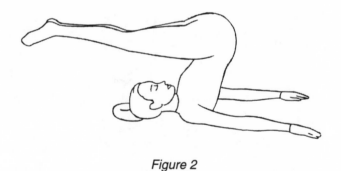

Figure 2

Figure 2. Bring your legs over your head as in the drawing. If your feet cannot be brought over to touch the floor, put pillows or a stool to your limit or bend your knees at your ears. Hold this pose for 20 seconds to 5 minutes.

Camel

The weight of the head in this pose, at least ten pounds, augments the toning and flexibility factors of this backward bending pose. As the muscles of the upper back contract to maintain the pose, the muscles across the chest are stretched and lengthened, improving circulation as well as toning and alignment.

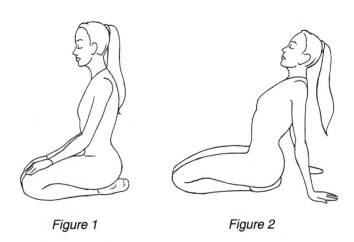

Figure 1   *Figure 2*

The Pose

Figure 1. Kneel with legs about six inches apart. Sitting on heels, lower shoulders and lift chest erect.

Figure 2–3. Place hands behind feet, lean back on arms and allow your head to drop back as you arch your back.

It aids in deep breathing, firms the waist and abdomen, tones the neck and throat.

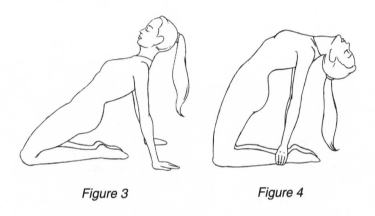

Figure 3   Figure 4

Figure 4. Place a hand on your heel, press the pelvis forward, and drop the head as you reach, stretch, and place the other hand on the other heel. Push the front of your body forward, placing your weight on your knees. Hold the pose, arching gently for several breaths; return one hand at a time to your thighs and relax.

LEARN HOW TO BELLY DANCE

I believe every woman, at one time or another, has been intrigued with the idea of belly dancing. Through the ancient art of belly dancing, you can tone, lose weight, and have a lot of fun.

If you find that you like belly dancing, I suggest you get yourself some Middle Eastern music and do the movements to the music. The same movements can be done to slow or fast music. You really should get the music, period. It will make it easier to get into it, blend the movements together, and dance. Dance in front of the mirror, so that you can see if you are doing it correctly. Tie a scarf around your hips and begin to move. Have fun with it!

I started belly dancing when I was twenty-three years old. I was three months pregnant, and I was very unhappy with my body. I went to the doctor and asked him what to do with the excess skin around my stomach from the pregnancy with my first child. I really wasn't in such bad shape, but I thought I was gross. He told me to get on some kind of program. I was afraid that I would try something for two weeks and quit, so he suggested that I take up belly dancing. He said it would help build my abdominal muscles, make childbirth easier, and would give me more control of my body. This sounded great to me.

I was on a journey. I had to find a belly dancer to teach me how to slither like a snake. I found a woman that had lived in Egypt for a while and was a professional belly dancer who danced at a local Greek restaurant, where she taught classes. She agreed to give me private lessons. I had so much fun, and it came so easily to me, that I danced the entire time I was pregnant.

Of course as my stomach grew, I slowed the movements down. I didn't throw my hips; I slowly moved them. I danced every day. I loved it. The music would get in my blood and I would start moving.

I was amazed; the day I gave birth to Heidi, I looked better than before I had gotten pregnant. I continued to dance for fun and exercise. Then I started teaching the dance, danced at a couple of Middle Eastern restaurants on occasion, and operated a business, *The Belly Telegram*, for a few years.

Twenty-three years have passed since I began belly dancing. I really don't do it often anymore, but I know the results are terrific and it is much fun. I dance on occasion when asked to, and every once in a while will teach a class.

Don't be shy; you can do it privately in your own home all by yourself. As you get into the music and start shaking and shimmying, you will melt the fat right off your body.

Arm Movements

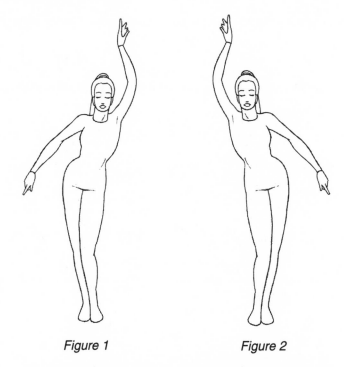

Figure 1   Figure 2

Figure 1. Lean back a little from your waist. Start with your right arm down as in the drawing, raising your left arm slowly. At the same time, bend your knees so that you can push your right hip toward your right arm.

Figure 2. Very slowly bring your left arm down, at the same time bringing your right arm up as it is extended out to the side of you.

You'll find that to push your hips from side to side as you are doing this, you will alternate bending your knees. Push your hips as far as you can from side to side.

At the same time that you push your hips to the right, pull in the left side of your stomach muscles and push out with the right side. When you go to the right side, push your muscles to the left. Sound hard? With leaning back a little, it will make it easier. Practice and don't give up—you will get it.

Develop Your Stomach Muscles

This is easy!

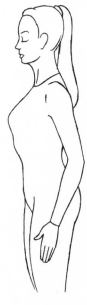

Figure 1

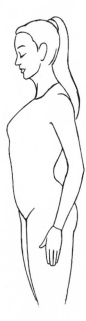

Figure 2

Figure 1. Pull your stomach in as far as you can. Feel the muscles up under your ribs being pulled.

Figure 2. Push out as far as you can. Lift your butt up some as you are doing this and remember to push out under the ribs as well.

Push out, hold; pull in and hold. Your holds should be for five seconds. Do this often, you can do it while doing the dishes, watching television, doing anything.

Doing this will help develop the abdominal muscles to help you control your abdomen while dancing.

Neck

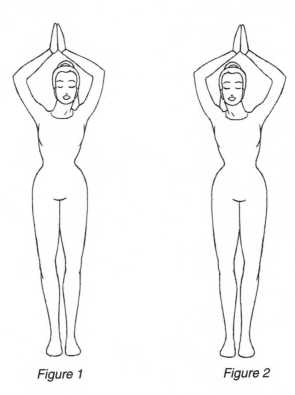

Figure 1   Figure 2

Figure 1. You can do this movement with your hands in the cobra position over your head as in the drawings, or in front of
your bust, with elbows extended out to your sides. Your hips
and legs should remain stationary.

Figure 2. Glide your head, keeping your face directed forward,
not turning it. Push your chin as far as you can to line your
head to the center of your breast, or as far as you can push it
without twisting or turning your head.

This is done very slowly, gliding back and forth. This is a great
exercise for the neck and chin.

Shoulders

Stand with your feet flat on the floor about six inches apart.

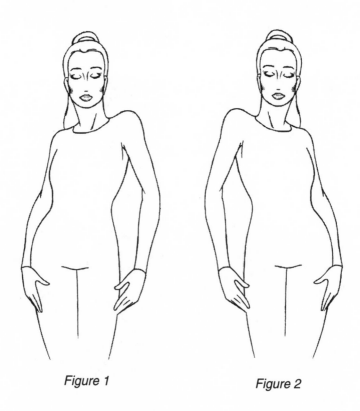

Figure 1   Figure 2

Figure 1. Drop your right shoulder as low as you can. At the same time that you drop the shoulder, take your left shoulder and in a circular motion bring it forward, up as far as you can and around to the back of you and down.

Figure 2. Repeat movement, dropping your left shoulder.

While you are doing this, slide your hips from side to side. As you get this down pat, put more body into it and really exaggerate the movements. This is done to very slow music.

The Camel Walk

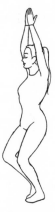

Figure 1

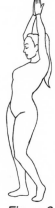

Figure 2

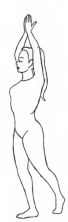

Figure 3

Figure 1. Stand with your feet together and knees slightly bent. Arms go up in the cobra position, with hands together.

Figure 2. Take a step with your right foot and pull your hips forward, leaving the top of your body behind as you make your body sway.

Figure 3. Pull the top part of your body forward as you take another step. Again, sway your body is you walk around. You should be slithering around slowly, dramatically, lifting and dropping your chest as you sway.

Hip Movements

Here is where you really start moving and shaking! We're going to start with some simple, basic hip movements.

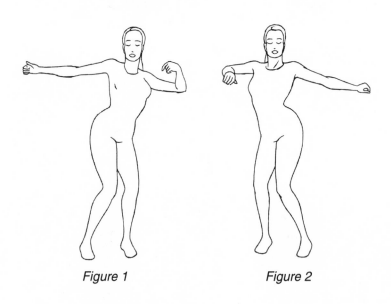

Figure 1   *Figure 2*

Thrusts

Your arms will be held out to the side while you do this, or alternate your arms as in the drawings.

Figure 1. Stand with your feet about eight inches apart. Try it—you may want to move your feet farther apart—whatever is most comfortable. Lean back a little. Swing your hips to the right.

Figure 2. Your knees will both be bent, one more so than the other. As if in an arch, throw your hip to the left. Your hip will actually make half a circle. You can do this with your feet flat on the floor or on your toes. Do what is most comfortable.

Sit and Kick and Its Variations

Basic Sit and Kick

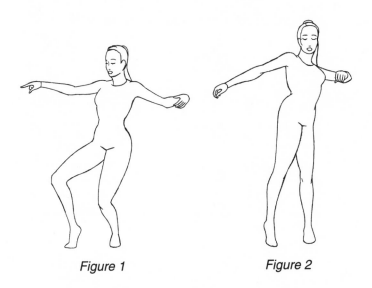

Figure 1   Figure 2

Figure 1. Put one foot flat on the floor. The other foot is a little bit ahead of you and you are on your toes. Lean back a little with arms out to the sides. Sit; drop your hips as though you were going to sit down; go as low as you can.

Figure 2. Swing your hip around and as high as you can. Your toes will be turning as though you are putting out a cigarette.

Again sit, and kick your hip out. Switch to the other hip and switch back and forth. You can do repetitions of five on one side and five on the other.

You can also sit and kick. The foot that is flat on the floor remains on the floor, but turns. You can sit kick, step with the toes, sit kick, and step. You will be going around in a circle with the one foot never leaving the floor, just turning with the rest of your body.

Sit, Sit, Sit, and Kick

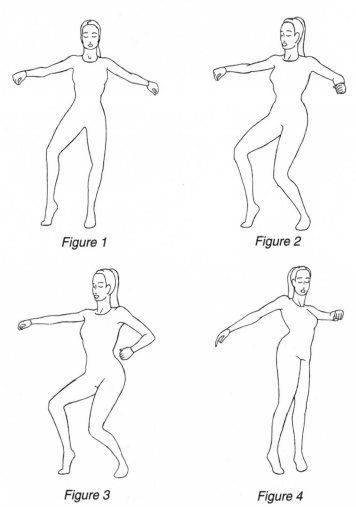

Figure 1

Figure 2

Figure 3

Figure 4

Figure 1. Stand flat on one foot, arms extended, right foot out on your toes. Lean back a little.

Figures 2 and 3. This time sit (drop your hips) just a little; drop again, sitting a little lower; then a third time, ouch!

Figure 4. Throw your hip out as far as you can.

You will sit, sit, sit, and kick.

Sit, Kick, and Walk

Okay, you have the sit and kick down.

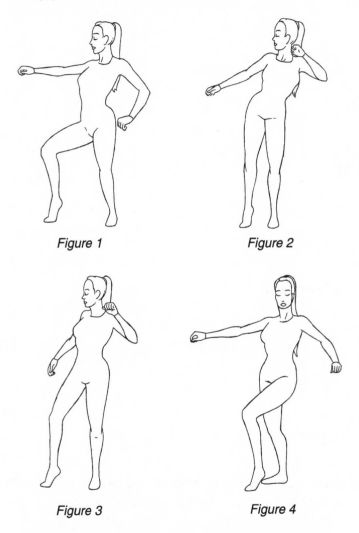

Figure 1

Figure 2

Figure 3

Figure 4

Figure 1. Put your left foot on the floor, your right toes are out.

Figure 2 and 3. Sit and kick, then with the right foot, step.

Figure 4. Put your right foot flat on the floor, left toes out, and go directly to a sit on the left side.

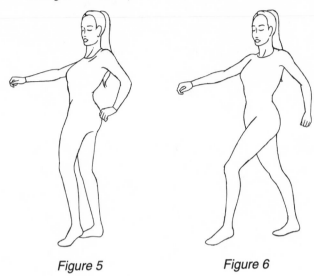

Figure 5   Figure 6

Figure 5 and 6. Kick the left hip, step with the left foot, going directly to the sit and kick of the other hip.

You will walk around the room in a circle, repeating sit, kick, and step.

Shimmy

You can't learn to belly dance without doing the shimmy. I didn't include a photo because you can't really show this in a picture unless it is a movie camera.

This is fun and easy once you get the knack of it.

Stand with your feet slightly apart and move your shoulders. Try variations until you've got it. One shoulder forward and at the same time your other shoulder should be going to the back of you. Do this until you have a momentum going; your breasts should be shimmying and shaking. You can walk around gracefully as you are doing this. When you have mastered this, try making a circle with your ribcage and at the same time continue shimmying.

Now for your hips. Stand with your feet about six inches apart. Relax your butt, take your knees and push one forward as you straighten the other one and alternate.

Do this quickly—faster—faster!

Your heinie should be a-wiggling and a-jiggling.

You've got it. Try walking around shimmying both your chest and your hips!

chapter 14

my final thoughts

I hope you go through this book and try different things. Do what you are attracted to. Do what feels right for you.

I hope this book makes an impact on your life, teaches you that you can control your thoughts, your body, your destiny.

I want you to say

I love myself.
I approve of myself.
I feed myself nourishing foods.
I will find fun ways to exercise.
I love lots of energy.
In my world, all is well. Everything is in divine order.

This book was meant for you, to awaken the possibilities within you, rejuvenate your body, mind, and soul to total balanced health. For you to have this, you must start today!

By making losing weight joyful, playful, and having a childlike state, you will have the best progress.

It has been proven that what you imagine right now will be what your life gives you in the future. You are in total control of your imagination. Use it wisely.

Having a childlike mind will bring the best results. Children don't think there are limits.

My heart goes out to you with nourishing, caring love for your total wellness!

references and resources

References and Suggested Reading Material

Barnes, Broda Otto, and Lawrence Galton. 1976. *Hypothyroidism: The Unsuspected Illness.* New York: HarperCollins Publishers, Incorporated.

Bell, Lorna, and Eudora Seyfer. 1990. *Gentle Yoga.* Berkeley, California: Celestial Arts

Bragg, Patricia, and Paul C. Bragg. 1999. *Apple Cider Vinegar: Miracle Health System.* Santa Barbara, California: Health Science.

Christopher, John R. *Mucusless Diet.* Springville, Utah: Bi World Industries, Incorporated.

Christopher, John R. 1991. *Dr. Christopher's Three-Day Cleansing Program.* Springville, Utah: Bi World Industries, Incorporated.

Christopher, John R., and Cathy Gileadi. 1994. *Every Womans Herbal.* Springville, Utah: Christopher Publications.

Crayhon, Robert, M.S. 1998. *The Carnitine Miracle: The Supernutrient Program That Promotes High Energy, Fat*

Burning, Heart Health, Brain Wellness, and Longevity. New York: M. Evans & Company, Incorporated.

Crayhon, Robert, M.S. 1996. *Robert Crayhon's Nutrition Made Simple: A Comprehensive Guide to the Latest Findings in Optimal Nutrition.* New York: M. Evans & Company, Incorporated.

Crook, William G., M.D. 1989. *The Yeast Connection Cookbook: A Guide to Good Nutrition and Better Health.* New York: Prof Bks F.

Crook, William G., M.D. 1997. *The Yeast Connection and the Woman.* New York: Prof Bks Future Heal.

Crook, William G., M.D. 1999. *The Yeast Connection Handbook.* New York: Prof Bks F.

Erdmann, Robert, and Meirion Jones. 1989. *The Amino Revolution.* New York: Simon & Schuster Trade.

Gittleman, Ann Louise. 1993. *Guess What Came to Dinner: Parasites and Your Health.* Wayne, New Jersey: Avery Publishing Group, Inc.

Hay, Louise L. 1988. *Heal Your Body: The Mental Causes for Physical Illness and the Metaphysical Way to Overcome Them.* Carlsbad, California: Hay House, Inc.

Hay, Louise L. 1987. *You Can Heal Your Life.* Carlsbad, California: Hay House, Inc.

Johnson, Debbie. 1997. *Think Yourself Thin: The Visualization Technique That Will Make You Lose Weight without Diet or Exercise.* New York: Hyperion.

Kroeger, Hanna. 1991. *Parasites: The Enemy Within.* Carlsbad, California: Hanna Kroeger Publications.

Langer, Stephen, M.D., and James F. Scheer. 1989. *Solved: The Riddle of Weight Loss.* Rochester, Vermont: Inner Traditions International, Limited.

Papon, R. Donald. *Homeopathy Made Simple 1999.* Charlottesville, Virginia: Hampton Roads Publishing Co. Inc.

Samskrti and Veda. 1977. *Hatha Yoga, Manual 1.* Honesdale, Pennsylvania: Glenview Himalayan International Institute.

Somers, Suzanne. 1997. *Suzanne Somers' Eat Great, Lose Weight.* New York: Crown Publishing Group.

Wallach, Joel. "Dead Doctors Don't Lie" audiocassettes.

Washburn, Loretta. 1994. *Mind Travelers: Portraits of Famous Psychics and Healers of Today.* Norfolk, Virginia: Hampton Roads Publishing Co.

Washburn, Loretta. 1997. *The Practical Art of Magick: Creating Your Own Reality* audiocassettes. Virginia Beach, Virginia: Loretta Washburn.

Resources

For more information on parasites, write to
  The Rheumatoid Disease Foundation
  Old Harding Rd.
  Franklin, TN 37064

For more information about yeast-related problems, contact
  The International Health Foundation
  P.O. Box 3494
  Jackson, TN 38303
This is a nonprofit organization and has helped thousands of people. Dr. William Crook is the founder. The foundation needs outside support and welcomes donations.

For homeopathy by mail, contact
  Dr. R. Donald Papon
  P.O. Box 52
  High Bridge, NJ 08829
  1-908-638-9963

To order the catalogue of herbs that Dr. John Christopher has
formulated, call or write
1-800-453-1406
Christopher Enterprises, Inc.
1195 Spring Creek Place
Springville, UT 84663-0777

To order *Dr. Christopher's Three Day Cleansing Program,
Mucusless Diet and Herbal Combinations*, call or write
1-800-372-8255
Christopher Publications
P.O. Box 412
Springville, UT 84663-0777
I highly recommend that you purchase this book, as I did not include all information you may want to know about.

For ordering DFH Discount Supplements, call 1-800-847-8302.

For authoritative information on garlic and other herbal medicines, contact
American Botanical Council
P.O. Box 201660
Austin, TX 78720
Fax: 512-231-1924.

To receive a catalogue from The Heritage Store, simply call
1-800-862-2923, which spelled out is 800-To Cayce.

For help locating herbs, contact
The Herb Finder
P.O. Box 2557
St. George, UT 84771-2557
801-652-9593

Index

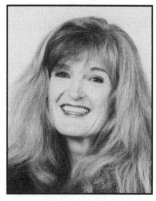
Bob Nielsen

about the author

Loretta lives in Norfolk, Virginia. She was born in Oakland, California, and has three grown daughters: Gerda, Heidi, and Shelly. The joy of her life is in spending it with her grandson, Mark.

She is the author of *Mind Travelers: Portraits of Famous Psychics and Healers of Today.* She also wrote and produced the audiocassettes *The Practical Art of Magick: Creating Your Own Reality.*

Loretta is also a photographer and exhibits her work all over the world in galleries and museums. As a health researcher, she can be heard on radio shows in this country, teaching people how to have optimal health, to live longer, and to change their lives forever for the better.

You can contact her by writing

Loretta Washburn
P.O. Box 3461
Virginia Beach, VA 23454

Hampton Roads Publishing Company

. . . for the evolving spirit

Hampton Roads Publishing Company
publishes books on a variety of subjects including
metaphysics, health, complementary medicine,
visionary fiction, and other related topics.

For a copy of our latest catalog,
call toll-free, 800-766-8009,
or send your name and address to:

Hampton Roads Publishing Company, Inc.
134 Burgess Lane
Charlottesville, VA 22902
e-mail: hrpc@hrpub.com
www.hrpub.com